Assertive Parenting

I0875926

If you want to discover the key elements for building a secure attachment with a child, you have come to the right book. Psychologist and psychotherapist Milena González presents the importance of learning to educate from a place of love that sustains, as well as limits that protect. In parenting, love and limits go hand in hand; they do not conflict with each other. Both are as necessary for a child's emotional health as food and sleep are for their physical health.

This book takes a comprehensive look at childhood and a compassionate view of those adults who, while not perfect, want to learn to see and treat the children in their lives with respect. All of this is done by deconstructing parenting models and patterns that affect not only the bond between parents and children, but also the mental health of the little ones.

Children construct an idea of themselves and the world around them based on the way they are viewed and treated by those who matter to them. To define themselves as capable or incapable, strong or weak, a failure or the opposite, they will draw on their emotional memory and remain faithful to the words, looks, and treatment they received mainly from those who defined them in their early years. It is never too late to learn to do things differently. By reading this book, you will discover how to improve relationships with children by building a secure attachment.

Milena González is a psychologist specializing in Trauma, Attachment, and Emotional Education. She completed a Master's Degree in Emotional Intelligence at the University of Valencia. She is an expert in brief psychotherapy with children and adolescents, and clinical and trauma intervention with EMDR. She has been certified as a Positive Discipline Educator for Families and in the Classroom by the Positive Discipline Association and the Spanish Association of Positive Discipline. In addition to her private practice, she teaches training courses in centers dedicated to promoting treatment of children and assertive parenting workshops for Spanish-speaking families and teachers. She also promotes assertive parenting through her social media accounts: @unamamapsicologa_.

Assertive Parenting

How to Build Secure Attachment and Care for Children's Mental Health

Milena González

Routledge
Taylor & Francis Group
NEW YORK AND LONDON

Designed cover image: Getty Images

First published in English 2027
by Routledge
605 Third Avenue, New York, NY 10158

and by Routledge
4 Park Square, Milton Park, Abingdon, Oxon, OX14 4RN

Routledge is an imprint of the Taylor & Francis Group, an informa business

Crianza Asertiva (3rd edition) by Milena González

ISBN: 978-1-041-32784-4 (hbk)
ISBN: 978-1-041-28043-9 (pbk)
ISBN: 978-1-003-78448-7 (ebk)

DOI: 10.4324/9781003784487

Typeset in Times New Roman
by codeMantra

Contents

Foreword

Dear reader, congratulations. You have, in your hands, a real treasure that will change your daily life with your children.

Whether they are your children, nieces and nephews, grandchildren, neighbors, students, or patients, the content of this book is so valuable for understanding them, relating to them, and accompanying them "as they weather the storm" (in the author's words) or storms of life, that it will become the one that replaces all others on your nightstand.

Assertive parenting is cause for celebration because there is no one better than Milena, a communicator par excellence, to explain it and spread the word.

The eight chapters that make up this book take us on a wonderful journey through the adventure of accompanying our children in their early years with the firm intention of helping them thrive while promoting their mental health. I can't think of a better project.

Milena turns us into "life coaches" and urges us to roll up our sleeves and embark on the task of building and cementing the foundations of what will become the resources our children will have at their disposal to face the challenges of the present and the future.

This book does not analyze the pandemic and its effects on children's mental health, but it does use the pandemic to illustrate and make us aware of the strong impact that social crises have on our children's health and the importance of committing ourselves to their well-being and resilience.

It breaks with the myth that raising children without shouting and a firm hand makes them "fragile," but it also does not agree with those who advocate for parenting without limits where anything goes. It advocates for assertiveness, a skill that we can train ourselves to have, and for encouraging rather than praising.

In addition, it explains in detail fundamental concepts such as those related to attachment, assertiveness, psychological trauma, emotions, and anxiety, immersing us in the wonderful world of understanding and interpreting our little ones ("bad behavior is a cry for help") and offering specific interventions for the most common conflict situations. The practical guidance on teaching life skills, which involves looking beyond the tip of the iceberg, beyond the behavior we observe, and the MAC method, which invites us to model, accompany, and channel, are good examples of these specific solutions.

Each chapter and each concept is thoroughly explained and illustrated with simple, everyday examples. It is clear that the author knows what she is talking about, as a mother, psychotherapist, and trainer.

I find particularly important the value given throughout this book (and especially in Chapter 4) to the perspective of caregivers, the distribution of places and roles in the family (according to Karpman's triangle: rescuer, persecutor, or victim), and the so-called Pygmalion effect. Milena does not forget how essential it is to contextualize children's development within a family system which, with its rules, permissions, and mandates, influences and even determines how their brains will be shaped and the rest of their development as people: how they see themselves (or do not), how they understand themselves and those with whom they interact, the narrative about themselves and the world, everything.

Begoña Aznárez

President of The Spanish Society of Psychosomatic Medicine and Psychotherapy (SEMPyP)

Acknowledgments

I thank God for knowing what it means to raise children and be a mother firsthand, and for accompanying and supporting me through my five pregnancies. Today, I have the joy of hearing three of them call me "mom," and I continue to embrace the other two in my heart.

To Andrés, my life partner and father of my children, for giving his all in his role as a dad and inspiring me every day to continue building a secure bond with our three little ones. I couldn't have anyone better by my side for this mission. I love you.

To Ana María, Gabriela, and Andrés, for helping me see beyond theory and "bad behavior" and teaching me to look at the human being in front of me from my own experience as a mother. You three are the best teachers I've ever had. I will always love you.

To Deborah Donda, manager of Lorelei Tarón, CEO and founder of Onthego Group, for teaching me that what we do goes beyond a dream or a goal. Thank you for constantly reminding me that all of this has to do with our essence and our purpose in life.

Many thanks to each of the families, children, and adolescents who have come into my life trusting that together we can work as a team. It is their stories that transform and challenge my life and help me grow as a professional and, above all, as a person.

Special thanks and warm regards to Begoña Aznárez and José Luis Marín, presidents of the Spanish Association of Psychosomatic Medicine and Psychotherapy. Much of what I know, what I teach in this book, and what I share as a mental health professional comes from what I have "drunk in" from them and their integrative model of psychotherapy, which has contributed to my personal and professional life. It is an honor to have them as teachers and to be part of the SEMPyP family. Begoña, I especially want to thank you for agreeing to write the foreword to my first book. I still can't believe it. I never tire of saying that you are the greatest psychologist and psychotherapist I have ever known and the one who has influenced me most professionally.

And I would also like to thank my inner child, whose story, fears, complexes, and pleasant and difficult moments have inspired much of the work I do on behalf of families and children.

AI usage statement

DeepL Pro was used to generate a draft translation from the Spanish edition. The text has been subsequently revised.

Chapter 1

Introduction

This book aims to answer a question that many of us who have the gift and responsibility of raising children often ask ourselves: What can I do to help my child thrive in life while promoting their mental health? If we think about it, this question focuses specifically on the fundamental role we have as caregivers in building and strengthening the necessary foundations that will serve as the basis for our children's mental health.

Now, this book may also be useful to those who do not have children but are in close or direct contact with them, and this is one of its main aims. This book is addressed primarily to parents and caregivers who are raising children. But, as mentioned above, the intention is to raise collective awareness about the importance of ensuring, as a society, the protection, care, safety, importance, and shelter that every child deserves and needs. This is a shared responsibility, whether or not we have children.

This book is not about COVID-19 and its consequences for children's mental health. It does, however, include specific references, especially in the first chapter, to emotional and social well-being, as it is one of the most challenging situations we are currently facing in terms of mental health. However, what you will read in both the first chapter and throughout the book is useful for any situation that has caused or may cause stress or anxiety in your child.

This book addresses the importance of positive treatment during childhood as a protective factor for mental health in children and adults, a concept that is discussed and developed throughout the book under the name of *assertive parenting.* By the end of the book, it is hoped that you will have developed greater awareness and sensitivity in order to:

1 accompany your children when they are going through difficult and traumatic moments, providing them with the necessary tools to integrate what they have experienced.
2 understand what trauma is and what can be done to prevent a situation with a high emotional impact from causing traumatic injury to your child.
3 use tools and resources that allow you to accompany them in their daily life, acting as the life coach your child needs while also building a secure bond with them.

DOI: 10.4324/9781003784487-1

1.1 A small warning

The content of this book may be uncomfortable for some readers, particularly those who:

1 believe that educating with affection and love will create a generation of "crystal children."
2 consider harsh discipline necessary and believe that a timely spanking never hurt anyone.
3 believe that assertive parenting means setting no limits and allowing children to do whatever they want.

Before you continue reading, I would like to clarify that I will generally use the word "child" to refer to both boys and girls. This avoids the need to constantly distinguish between them, which can slow down the reading. Similarly, at different points in the book, I will use the words "caregiver" or "caregivers" to refer to father, mother, or the person responsible for the child's care.

Furthermore, I would also like to thank you for taking the time to read this book.

I sincerely hope that everything I discuss here will help you in the important task of educating your child and that you will be able to do so in a more conscious, assertive, and meaningful way for both you and your child.

Chapter 2

Let's talk about children's mental health

> We define mental health as the harmonious and continuous progression between these two extremes (chaos-rigidity). By helping our children connect their left and right sides, we give them a better chance of avoiding the extremes of chaos and rigidity, and live in the flexible stream of mental health.
>
> (Daniel Siegel and Tina Bryson)

Between 10% and 20% of all children worldwide experience some form of mental health problem.[1]

This information is not new to us, and it seems clear that since the pandemic began, there has been greater awareness of its effects, not only on physical health but—above all—also on mental health, especially in our children and adolescents. No one expected what we are going through, and I believe that even though time has passed, we still cannot imagine the consequences that this whole situation has had on mental health.

We live in an increasingly unpredictable society marked by uncertainty. We are often surrounded by talks of wars, social, family, economic, and all kinds of crises. The question that has been circulating for years is usually: "What happens next?"

We often talk about the political and economic consequences of crises. One day it may be a health crisis; another day, it might be something else. Yet, without realizing it, each crisis gives rise to and spreads other difficult situations that directly affect mental health. These effects may be less visible and more silent, but they are so persistent that they make no distinction between adults, young people, and children. Crises, including health crises, can generate anxiety, stress, and the feeling of helplessness when we are unable to change the situations that affect us or return to who we were before.

We have always been required a society, an educated and informed society, that is committed to children's mental health, and can optimally help and support the younger generations.

DOI: 10.4324/9781003784487-2

Did you know?

A study conducted by the University of Ottawa[2] states that anxiety, along with post-traumatic stress disorder and depression, has increased exponentially in the global population, with anxiety becoming up to four times more common than before the pandemic.

If adults were so emotionally affected by the health crisis and everything that came with it, can you imagine how a child's inner world is shaken by situations of uncertainty, stress, worry, or anxiety?

The United Nations has indicated that the COVID-19 pandemic and its consequences have not only compromised our physical health but also affected our mental health, particularly that of the most vulnerable people, including children and adolescents.[3]

Let's start with the fact that it is difficult for children, due to their cognitive development and brain immaturity, to explain in their own words what they are experiencing, feeling, and what is causing them internal or emotional discomfort. This is why the presence of an attuned adult is important in a child's life: an adult who can help the child feel understood; translate all their internal emotional experiences; and express their fears, anxieties, worries, doubts, and uncertainties into words.

We must learn to see children beyond their behavior. We need to understand that feeling of suffocation, a headache, an almost daily complaint of a stomach-ache, difficulty falling asleep, and the repeated lack of appetite at mealtimes may be their way of asking for help and telling us that something inside them is not working properly. Instead of dismissing these symptoms as childish things that will pass, our role in caring for children's mental health is to train ourselves as life educators, so that we can attend their emotions and feelings with the same diligence and urgency that we show when they have a physical injury.

The demand for the treatment of childhood anxiety, behavioral problems, inattention, sleep disorders, and mood disorders has increased dramatically since the pandemic began. Caring for health in childhood is an investment we make today, with short-, medium-, and long-term effects.

But what do we mean when we talk about mental health? This will be explained in the next section.

2.1 What is mental health and how has it been affected in recent years?

The World Health Organization (WHO) states that "health is a state of complete physical, mental, and social well-being, and not merely the absence of disease or infirmity."[4]

I would like to call it "the tripod of mental health."

This definition clearly reflects the importance of emphasizing the mental, emotional, and social aspects of human beings and not just one part of them (physical), as we usually tend to do.

A mother might say, "The truth is that Pedro hasn't been affected by his grandfather's death as much as I thought he would be, because he hasn't lost his appetite and continues to eat as usual. In fact, at his last checkup, the pediatrician told me he's very healthy." We have traditionally understood health almost exclusively in physical terms: "if you're not sick, you're fine." However, the WHO itself insists that there is no health without mental health.

In this sense, when we talk about the importance of optimal mental health in children, we are, of course, referring to their physical health, but also to their emotional, mental, and social well-being. In other words, we are referring to what I call their "Well-being."

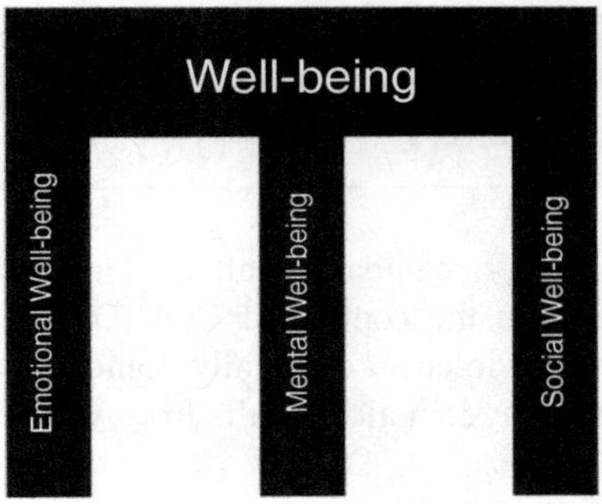

Ensuring this triad of "WELL-BEING" is the responsibility and obligation of governments, including parents, teachers, the scientific community, and health professionals.

Highly recognized associations backed by scientific evidence, such as the Platform of Associations of Psychiatry and Clinical Psychology for Child and Adolescent Mental Health in Spain, reported in a 2020 study on the widespread direct and indirect psychological and social effects of the pandemic, which could affect mental health both now and in the future. Therefore, although the health crisis we experienced a few years ago now seems like a thing of the past, its consequences for mental health are not over, and its psychological effects could even be passed from one generation to the next.

A report[5] submitted by the United Nations on a population study in Spain and Italy, involving 1,143 people between the ages of 18 and 66, showed that 85.7% observed changes in their children's emotional state and behavior during quarantine.

I am sure that you did not need to know about this study beforehand to recognize this reality. We experience this evidence every day in our homes, at work, in schools, and in public places. We notice that people are more stressed, irritable, sleepless, anxious, unfocused, exhausted, distant from others, and that they generally exhibit behaviors that reflect the emotional and psychological consequences of social crises or crises of any kind.

2.2 Social crises as a possible traumatic factor for the mental health of children and families

I don't know at what point in your life you are reading this. I don't know if it has been a few years or many years and it may sound obsolete to you; in fact, you don't have to read this to understand the rest of the book. But I want to make sure that, even as the years go by and the pandemic is a thing of the past, we don't forget what our children have gone through emotionally during this crisis. It's easy to forget, silence, and even minimize the moments of distress and uncertainty that we all experienced during those times, especially children.

> Did you know that studies show that violence against women and children had also increased during the pandemic?

UN Women carried out a campaign called "The pandemic in the shadows. Violence against women in the context of COVID-19,"[6] in which it warned of an increase in all types of violence, especially domestic violence, against women and girls. In the United Kingdom alone, calls from victims increased by 65% in a single week.

Many children were confined with abusive caregivers, living in daily fear of domestic and gender-based violence. There were families with children with disabilities or special needs who had no possibility of continuing to receive support, either for the children or for their caregivers.

Restrictions on movement, empty public spaces, economic, health, and safety concerns, and being isolated with abusers were factors that made life worse in all areas for many women, girls, and boys.

A survey conducted by Ipsos during the lockdown period reported widespread concern among the population about the psychological impact of both confinement and social distancing. Of the 13,785 adults surveyed between March 26 and 30, 2020, from 15 different countries, the majority responded that what concerned them most were the weakest and most vulnerable people, including children.

We mentioned earlier that optimal mental health must be guaranteed by complete emotional, mental, and social well-being. However, during that health crisis, it was clear that this concept was very well written on paper, but in reality we saw something very different.

John Bowlby, father of attachment theory, stated that mental health involves the successful management of conflicts, the universal conflict being to experience a desire and its opposite at the same time. I usually explain this concept to my three children as I learned it from my teacher Begoña Aznárez, president of the Spanish Association of Psychosomatic Medicine and Psychotherapy. Successfully managing the experience of a desire and its opposite at the same time is like strongly wanting to eat the ice cream you are holding while also not wanting to eat it because you don't want it to run out. There are two opposite desires!

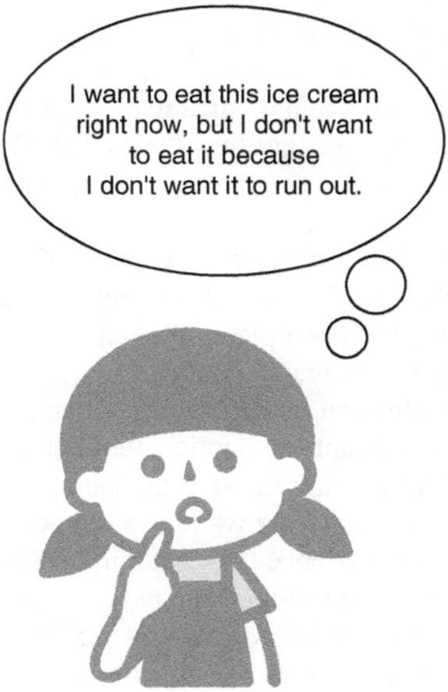

I want to eat this ice cream right now, but I don't want to eat it because I don't want it to run out.

Life isn't like ice cream, I know; sometimes it's more like not even having the slightest chance of getting that ice cream. And yet, if we stop thinking about it, this too is a conflict that needs to be resolved. Because the conflict usually arises when we turn a desire into a need.

The problem we faced during the pandemic was that many of our children were not simply dealing with desires—which are legitimate in themselves—but with unmet needs. What they were often asking for, sometimes through disruptive behavior, was help in meeting those needs. One example was their social and emotional need to play with friends in the park when this was not possible. How could we support them in a situation beyond our control? More broadly, how can we adequately support children when unwanted events occur—for example, when a loved one dies, they are separated from someone they love, or plans unexpectedly fall through?

Well, Bowlby also argued that mental health is the successful management of conflicts and this task cannot be performed by the child alone. Children are dependent beings, and they need a secure base from which they can learn to look at themselves and the world around them: a base from which they can generate models of thinking and patterns of functioning; a secure base to which they can turn without fear when life outside causes fear; and a base they can trust, knowing that from there they can see themselves as someone capable of asking for help when they need it because they have someone capable of providing it when they need it.

It is clear that the pandemic made things difficult for all of us who lived through it, and yet we were not all treated equally. We made our children "invisible" in many ways and forced them to act as if nothing was happening, even though their whole world around them had changed drastically. Their routines changed, as did the way they interacted with their families, their educational models, their leisure time, and the possibility of talking about their fears, their frustration, anger, and sadness.

One way to silence their inner world, and possibly with the noblest of intentions, was to reward them for their resilience and call them heroes. As if that gave them a voice and provided them with a complete, integrated, effective, and coherent narrative of what they were experiencing.

Constantly describing children as naturally resilient, calling them heroes, and emphasizing how well they adapt to chaotic situations is not necessarily the best way to care for them. Many children were not being resilient; they were being forced to adapt without understanding what was happening or having a complete account of what they had experienced. Developing resilience is not the same as being compelled to adjust. As neurologist and psychiatrist Boris Cyrulnik explains, protective adaptation is not always evidence of resilience. He defines resilience as the ability to face life's adversities and transform pain into a driving force for growth.

Developing the flexibility that builds resilience requires support, attunement, and physical and emotional safety. Without these, you can survive, but you won't emerge stronger.

We have often witnessed the implementation of measures that ignore the needs of the most vulnerable. From the outset, the harshest measures were taken with regard to children. Caregivers found it extremely difficult to meet their children's basic needs. Children were unable not only to meet in person, as the situation obviously required, but also to access the technology needed to stay in touch, even if only online, and to see their loved ones.

These were important aspects of their lives. To this we must add the stress of not being able to attend virtual classes because, incidentally, teachers were required and overburdened with the obligation to continue teaching their classes as if nothing had happened.

Ensuring children's mental health was not a priority for administrative and judicial bodies, partly because families were not a priority on the political agenda. Neglecting families means neglecting children. While we saw borders gradually opening up for tourists, bars slowly filling to capacity, roads becoming a little busier every day, permission being granted to go without masks outdoors, and stadiums once again filled with fans, we saw the opposite side of the coin in harsh restrictions on schools, a return to school without adequate rights and equity, and caregivers trying to balance work and family life.

Families and professionals had to repeatedly speak up to ensure that their rights were respected, that everyone's safety was guaranteed, and, ultimately, that the best interests of every child were taken into account, especially those children who have suffered the most in terms of education due to their parents' economic and social circumstances. For this reason, some NGOs, such as Save the Children, called on state and regional governments to invest in education to ensure a safe and inclusive return to the classroom.

Reflecting on children's mental health means rethinking what we have done in the past and what we are doing today as a society, as well as the model we are building. While it is true that many of us feel helpless when it comes to our legal system in terms of rights, it is also true that every adult has an individual responsibility toward children. If the pandemic has not helped us to reorganize our priorities, then what else do we have to experience as a society?

What is the message we have conveyed to our children and adolescents? What are the values, principles, and realities we are transmitting even now that the pandemic no longer poses a health threat?

A study conducted by the Child Mind Institute[7] (2021) revealed that one of the biggest concerns for adolescents throughout the pandemic was "falling behind academically."

As a mental health professional, this information has led me to question the implicit message we as a society are sending to our children and young people over the years. We continue to prioritize cognitive and academic skills over social and emotional ones, even though our daily experiences show us the state of our mental health.

Today more than ever, there is a clear need to invest in education and work together on behalf of children, in order to ensure mental health that enables not only physical well-being, but also emotional and social well-being.

2.3 Childhood fear and anxiety in difficult situations

As we will see throughout the book, our behavior is directly related to how we perceive and interpret the world around us. All behavior communicates an unmet need. This need may be physical; for example, when a child cries or complains because they are hungry or sleepy; it may also be social, as when you see your little one talking, eating, or sharing similar tastes with their friends. This behavior is related to the need to belong and feel part of the group. There may be cognitive needs as well; for example, when a child shows curiosity and wants to discover for themselves why their mother or teacher insists that they should not go near the electrical outlet in front of them but still tries to stick a fork in it to see what happens. But there are also emotional needs, and these are possibly the ones we find most difficult to address because they are the ones with which we are least familiar. It is easy for us to invest time in teaching our children to skate, ride a bike, do arithmetic, or read. And yet, we find it much more difficult to accompany, support, or empathize with our children's pain, frustration, anger, or sadness. I am convinced that you have a deep desire to do so, and yet when you find yourself in that situation, you may feel as overwhelmed as, or even more overwhelmed than, your child. That doesn't make you a terrible caregiver; you are doing the best you can with the tools you have.

It is impossible to hold a conversation in another language if no one has first taken the time to teach us that language. No matter how much we want to speak it, we lack the ability to do so. The good news is that we can learn it. Emotional language can also be taught, developed, and learned with a great deal of acceptance of our current reality, forgiveness for the mistakes we have made so far, compassion when we realize that we will continue to make mistakes, and enthusiasm when we realize that all new knowledge adds to our work as parents in terms of the emotional bond with our children.

And what does this have to do with the title of this section?

When we learn to see our children's needs, behavior, and emotional world from the perspective of the development and functioning of their immature brains, many of the loose ends we have regarding what it means to raise, accompany, validate, support, and empathize with them will start to "fall into place," making it much easier for us to help them in difficult situations. To stop seeing a child as "the fearful one" or "the anxious one" and to begin seeing them as a child with an emotional need to feel accompanied by an adult who explains and puts meaningful words to what is happening are two completely different things.

Let's get specific. To understand the child's brain and its influence on the child's behavior, especially in difficult, stressful, or uncertain situations, I'm going to explain it to you as I do with the families I work with. In the following chapters, we will also expand on the relationship between the child's brain and what we have mistakenly called "bad behavior" for years.

Let's start by imagining the brain as if it were divided into three parts, each representing a center with different functions: the lowest part, known as the "reptilian brain" and composed mainly of the brain stem and cerebellum, is responsible for keeping us safe. It specializes in instincts and is responsible for our bodily movements, breathing, digestion, sleep, and wakefulness. This brain center is known as the "survival center." It does everything possible to keep us alive.

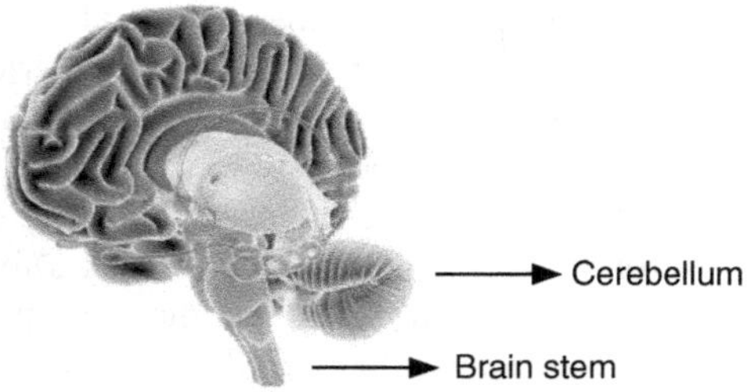

There is a second "command center," known as the "limbic brain" or "emotional brain." It is composed of key structures called "amygdalae," but also important structures such as the thalamus, hypothalamus, and hippocampus. In simple terms, this command center, which we share with mammals, aims to connect us emotionally with others. Therefore, it would be our affective or emotional center.

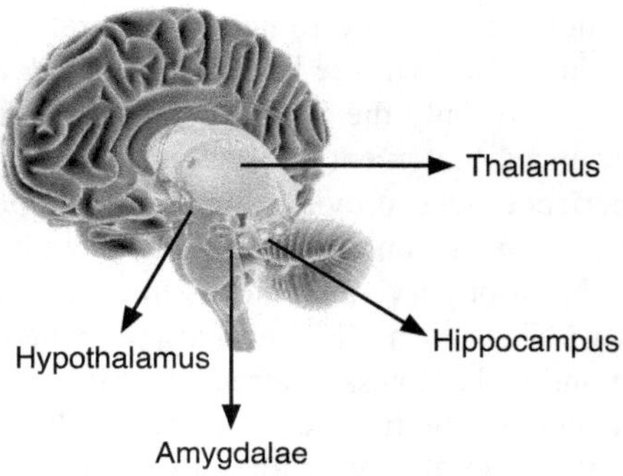

And finally, we have a third brain center composed of the neocortex, also called the "cerebral cortex," located behind our forehead. This is the last center to mature. It matures between the ages of 25 and 30, while the first two centers, survival and emotional centers, are formed when the child is born. From the neocortex, we make logical decisions, put ourselves in other people's shoes, plan, and anticipate; that is, we process information in a complex and cognitive way. Therefore, we know this center as the "higher center" or "executive center."

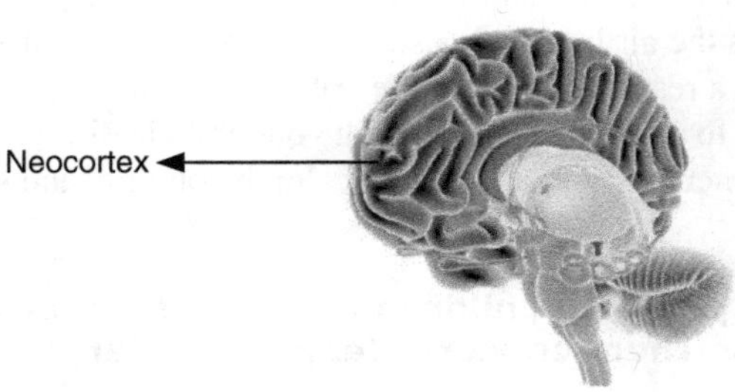

Therefore, we have three brain centers or "triune brain," as Paul MacLean called it in the 1980s. Among these three centers, one responsible for our survival, the second is responsible for our affective and emotional life, and the third is responsible for our more executive functions. Each of them has a specific way of helping us perceive, interpret, and explain the world around us. The first will lead us to perceive and explain what has happened to us in a more instinctive and visceral way, the second will do so in a more emotional way, and the third in a more cognitive way. None is better than the other; we need all three. Ideally, these centers should work as a team or, as Daniel Siegel calls it, work in an integrated way. But this is not always the case.

When a child finds themselves in a difficult situation and perceives any sign of insecurity or threat, their survival center is activated; their reptilian brain, responsible for keeping them safe, will put them into fight, flight, or freeze mode. It is not necessary to have a ferocious bear in front of them for this survival center to be activated; it is enough for the child to perceive threat and loneliness for their reptilian brain to kick in. As we will see later when we talk about trauma, what is traumatic for a person is not only the event itself, but the loneliness with which that person has experienced that event. Not having someone close to them who legitimizes their experience, who provides emotional support, who is a reliable place where that person feels safe and secure talking about it and thinking about it.

When the reptilian brain or survival center is in charge, the executive area of the brain "shuts down." That is why it is normal that, when the area of the brain responsible for sleep and wakefulness is affected, children may have more difficulty falling asleep, experiencing night terrors, or even shows signs of regression. For example, a child who had already learned to urinate or defecate in the toilet may suddenly start having accidents again.

Moreover, we may also find them more sensitive, irritable, lacking in appetite, or exhibiting a series of behaviors that, rather than being simple misbehavior, are the only way they have found to communicate their emotional distress to us.

Keep this in mind when faced with difficult situations, children do not have the brain maturity, vocabulary, or ability to reason about why they behave the way they do. They simply behave according to how they feel. Do not expect them to say, "Mom, the death of my pet has affected me so much that it has disrupted my nervous system to such an extent that I can't even sleep." And don't expect them to be aware that perhaps the birth of their sister has made them feel that they are "losing your love" and, as a result, they cry more, bite, and even hit themselves.

It is your ability to connect and bond with your child in difficult times that makes them feel secure, increasing their sense of calm, belonging, and safety.

2.4 How can you help children in difficult situations that cause them concern, fear, or anxiety?

In any stressful situation or when faced with news that changes the family dynamic, always keep this in mind: children are not scared by knowing what is happening; children are scared by not knowing what is happening. Let's start from the fact that children are constantly forming beliefs about themselves and the world around them. When they don't have information or perceive that it is being hidden from them, they will draw their own conclusions about what is happening around them. This is not ideal, because

Children have immature, egocentric, literal, and magical brains. These "ingredients" together, without the optimal narrative provided by their attachment figures, will end up generating beliefs, conclusions, and misconceptions that will impact their emotional well-being.

So let's do what we know is important, healthy, and appropriate for our children: communicate transparently. They don't need us to change the situation; they need certainty, to know that we are accessible no matter what happens, that we are sincere in telling them what we know and what we don't know, and above all, that we allow them to express their emotions without minimizing, censoring, distracting, or punishing them. I'll summarize this in four points:

1 Be honest and direct.
2 Create spaces where they can talk about how they feel, validating all emotions.
3 Provide reassurance.
4 Remember that your job is to accompany your child by offering your presence, not by eliminating their frustration.

We could summarize it like this:

"I would like us to talk about what is happening and what you have heard your friends and the news saying. Everything that is happening can make us feel scared and even angry because we cannot change it. Some of the plans and activities we had planned have had to be canceled. It's normal to feel angry or sad. And I want you to know that you can always come to me to tell me how you feel and what you think. I will do everything I can to keep us safe and get us through this together."

Notes

1 UNICEF. (2020). "Operational guidelines. Community-based mental health and psychosocial support in humanitarian settings: three-tiered support for children and families."
2 Mary, C., Blais-Rochette, C., Kokou-Kpolou, C., et al. (2021). "Prevalence of symptoms of depression, anxiety, insomnia, posttraumatic stress disorder, and psychological distress among populations affected by the COVID-19 pandemic: A systematic review and meta-analysis." *Psychiatry Research* 295, pp. 1–16.
3 UNICEF Spain. (2020). "Mental health and childhood in the context of COVID-19. Proposals from UNICEF Spain." June 2020. Available at: https://www.unicef.es/publicacion/salud-mental-e-infancia-en-el-escenario-de-la-covid-19-propuestas-de-unicef-espana
4 World Health Organization. (2022). "Mental health: strengthening our response." June 17, 2022. Available at: https://www.who.int/es/news-room/fact-sheets/detail/mental-health-strengthening-our-response
5 Orgiles, M., Morales, A., Delvecchio, E., Mazzeschi, C., and Espada, J. P. "Immediate psychological effects of the COVID-19 quarantine in youth from Italy and Spain" (Internet). *PsyArXiv*; Apr. 2020 (cited April 23, 2020). Available at: https://osf.io/5bpfz
6 UN Women. "The pandemic in the shadows. Violence against women in the context of COVID-19." Available at: https://www.unwomen.org/es/news/in-focus/ in-focus-gender-equality-in-covid-19-response/violence-against-women-during-covid-19
7 Osgood, K., Sheldon-Dean, H., and Kimball, H. (2021). "2021 Children's Mental Health Report: What we know about the COVID-19 pandemic's impact on children's mental health: and what we don't know." Child Mind Institute.

Chapter 3

Assertive parenting as the basis for protecting children's mental health

> While entire libraries have been written about mental illness, there are few definitions of mental health.
>
> (Siegel and Bryson)

Let us remember that, when we talk about mental health, according to the WHO, we are talking not only about the absence of diseases and conditions but also about emotional, psychological, and social well-being. In other words, promoting children's mental health means working toward a balance that allows children to develop their social and emotional skills while equipping them with the resources to face their daily challenges, based on the feeling that they are capable of asking for help when they need it and, at the same time, knowing that they have at least one adult they can ask for help.

At the beginning of this book, we said that one of the questions parents often ask themselves is what we can do to help their children thrive in life while promoting their mental health. Perhaps we don't ask ourselves this question in precisely these words. In more everyday language, it might be expressed as follows: "What can I do to make my child a good person?"

The answer to this question can be as simple as it is broad and complex: *we must treat our sons and daughters well*. But what does treating them well mean?

I would like to define it, as could not be otherwise, by referring to the concept that Jorge Barudy and Maryorie Dantagnan put forward in this regard: "Treating a child well means trying to offer them consistent communication in which there is agreement between what is said—the words—and the gestures, tone of voice, and body language."[1]

Consistency, in addition to being a basic parameter for fostering secure attachment with our children, is also a daily challenge for those of us who want to raise our children consciously, since many of us come from adult-centered family and social environments where our own voices may have been silenced, often by our own primary attachment figures.

DOI: 10.4324/9781003784487-3

> Each of us has developed our own concept of what it means to treat someone well based on our own life experiences, but, even more so, we have formed an idea of what it means to treat a child well based on our own experiences and the treatment we received in our own childhood.

In general, it seems that mothers and fathers agree when we say that everything we do is because we want the best for our children; there is usually no disagreement on this point. It is not common to hear a parent say, "The way I treat my child is so that they will have a worse life than I have."

However, while understanding the genuine desire to want the best for our children, many people have a predetermined and generalized idea about what it means to treat a child well and why they do so. This preconceived belief shapes the way caregivers relate to their children and the tools they use to help them succeed in life.

For some, treating a child well means providing security, support, emotional support, setting clear boundaries, and becoming what John Bowlby (1989)[2] called a secure base. For others, treating children well primarily has a starting point that usually goes something like "I'm doing this for your own good," and under this idea, physical punishment, verbal or psychological abuse, as well as indifference or isolation, can be used with the idea that this is how you are turning them into a good person.

These methods of viewing the good treatment of children have often generated heated debates among parents, teachers, pediatricians, and psychologists for centuries. They often come up in conversations we have at family gatherings, in parent–teacher conferences, in parenting workshops, in religious counseling, and even in children's literature. Parents and caregivers have access to thousands of books in different languages, written from these two perspectives on what good treatment means and, in general, what it means to raise children for life.

You've probably heard the saying, "I was beaten and I turned out fine." This belief largely indicates the state of our Western society. A society obsessed with visible behavior (what we do and don't do) and neglecting what really matters (who we are and how we feel).

Talking about the importance of treating children well goes beyond doing so "for their own good" or so that they grow up to be wonderful adults. We promote parenting based on mutual respect primarily because children and adolescents are human beings with rights,[3] not because we want them to "turn out" well or badly, as though they were a crop of cassava, bananas, or potatoes. We treat our children well because, first and foremost, they are human beings. Treating a child well means, first and foremost, treating them with kindness and respect for the simple fact that they are a person worth treating well.

> The level of good treatment toward anyone in the world does not depend on their height. Just because our child or student is shorter than us does not mean they are inferior.

Rudolf Dreikurs put it this way: "The right way to treat children is identical to the right way to treat our neighbors."[4]

Once we have assimilated these concepts, we can begin to look at our own life story with greater compassion and learn to reframe it. So, instead of saying, "I am who I am because of the beatings I received," we can reframe this narrative in a more adaptive way: "I am who I am despite the physical and emotional pain caused by the beatings I received."

Does this mean that assertive parenting is synonymous with being a completely healthy parent who never has emotional outbursts?

My answer is a resounding no. When it comes to parenting, one thing is certain: we are going to make mistakes. Therefore, when we talk about educating based on assertive parenting, we are not saying that we have to be perfect parents or caregivers who never make mistakes. In fact, making mistakes will be essential to teaching our children that mistakes are a great learning opportunity and part of life itself. When we make mistakes, we look for solutions instead of looking for and finding someone to blame. That is why another verb that should be unavoidable in parenting, and which I intend to convey to you throughout this book, is to repair. The power of repair is as important as it is essential in conveying our children the idea that others deserve to be respected and that, above all, they are people worthy of being treated with respect.

Let your child grow up with the certainty that when they make a mistake, they have made an error rather than feeling and assuming that they are the error.

Siegel and Bryson[5] say that we are human. There is no such thing as a perfect parent. But if we model how to deal with our mistakes and then repair the relationship, even our imperfect responses to misbehavior can be valuable and provide children with opportunities to face difficult situations and, as a result, help them in develop new skills.

I am aware that what you are reading sounds easy on paper and that the reality of parenting sometimes overwhelms us in our daily lives. It is exhausting, frustrating, and tiring to deal with the glass of milk that spills just before leaving the house, the lack of cooperation when it comes to brushing teeth, putting on shoes, getting dressed, showering, or going to bed. It hurts to feel powerless and yet still be responsible for empathetically accompanying the screams and tears caused perhaps because their sibling just hit them, and other times because we were the ones who caused that emotional pain. And it is precisely these kinds of daily interactions with our children that lead us to ask ourselves: am I hurting my child through the way I am raising them?

Am I giving them what they need to become a capable adult?

How can I apply discipline that educates them not only for the moment but for life? You want to foster an assertive education that promotes that secure bond in your relationship with your child, and at the same time, you want to reduce those tensed and stressed moments to promote their emotional and psychological well-being. Want me to tell you something? It's possible.

In fact, this is one of my main aims in writing this book. The goal is to introduce you to assertive parenting as a way of educating children in two directions: for the moment (gaining your children's cooperation while strengthening your relationship with them) and for the future (equipping them with the emotional resources they will need as adults). And why did I set these two goals? First, because I am a mother of three and I know what it is like to raise children, often feeling uncertain about whether what you are doing is helping your child. For more than 15 years, I have been going into classrooms and listening to stories from children and teenagers who deeply love their parents but who, at the same time, feel emotionally disconnected from them and, as a result, show changes in their behavior. Second, because in addition to being a mother, I am a psychologist and psychotherapist, and every day I receive messages from adults, especially mothers (it seems that socially women are allowed to appear more vulnerable than men), who tell me how the impact of their childhood experiences still affects them today.

> Treating our children with the same respect we would treat anyone else, knowing and responding to their needs, and helping them create a model of a respectful, kind, and pleasant world is a gift we give them for life.

It is important to keep in mind that our kindness, warmth, empathy, and love in our interactions with our children will be their first introduction to what it means to treat others well, and that these qualities will, in turn, become scaffolding on which they build their entire lives.

Our children will use their relationship with us as a reference point for forming an idea of what the world is like. As caregivers, our responsibility is to help make that world feel kind, pleasant, and trustworthy.

3.1 What is assertive parenting?

I want to start by sharing the same message I try to convey to families when I give talks or workshops on parenting: to fulfill your role as a mother or father through assertive parenting, you don't need to be perfect. You don't even have to get a little closer to being the ideal mom or dad. You don't have to have all the answers for every challenge and developmental stage your children go through. You don't have to have read all the parenting books or attended the hundreds of workshops recommended by the accounts you follow on social media. I haven't read them all either; honestly, I wouldn't have time for that.

Assertive parenting is not for a particular group of people; it is for imperfect parents like us who have a deep desire to raise our children, have a desire to become those adults that we ourselves may have needed when we were children.

The concept of assertiveness is one that has always struck me as very powerful ever since I discovered what it means, and I want to explain it briefly before we continue looking at what assertive parenting consists of. When we understand the importance of being assertive and how we integrate assertiveness into parenting, then the decisions we make when raising our children tend to be more intentional and conscious.

I would like to define assertiveness as a trainable skill—a skill that can be learned. In other words, we are not born assertive, but we can and—as caregivers—we must practice assertiveness.

And what do we train specifically? The ability to communicate what we think without stepping on others, hurting them, or stepping on ourselves, invalidating ourselves, and disrespecting our own boundaries. And this is precisely where our language and words play a very important role when we communicate with others. Because when we communicate with others and vice versa, it is not only what we say that matters, but also how we say it, when we say it, and to whom we say it. Our words carry significant emotional weight.

We tend to communicate in three basic styles: aggressive, passive, or assertive. There is also present a passive-aggressive style, which generally takes two forms: the person who is aggressive but hides it by making you doubt your own feelings or ideas and even making you feel guilty, and the person who tends to keep quiet and bottle things up and then at a certain point "explodes" and aggressively lets out all their anger. At this point, I will address those three communication styles: aggressive, passive, and assertive.

To illustrate what I am saying and the difference between one way of communicating and another, let's think about a 5-year-old girl—named Sofia—and the moment she has to return home after spending time with her best friend.

A mother who usually communicates aggressively will tell Sofia bluntly that it is time to go home. The girl starts to cry, looks at her and says she doesn't want to leave, that it's unfair because she hasn't visited her friend's house for many days and has not even been there very long, although we all know that they've spent the whole afternoon playing.

The mother, in an attempt to get her daughter to obey her, tells her that it's okay, that tomorrow they will come back for a little while after school. The girl, who is not very convinced, refuses to leave and cries even harder, shouting that she is the worst mother in the world. So this time, the mother, who is quite angry, tells her that if she had known she was going to make such a fuss, they would never have gone to her friend's house.

Annoyed, uncomfortable, and embarrassed in front of Sofia's friend's mother, she takes her daughter by force, thinking that this cannot be unaddressed and that Sofia needs to learn the hard way. If this is how she is at 5, what will she be like when she is 15? So, as soon as they walk out the door, she slaps Sofia on the butt and tells her that she doesn't care if she cries, but that from now on, she is grounded and cannot go back to her friend's house for at least a month, even though this mother knows how difficult it is to stick to that punishment because going to Sofia's friend's house is also a break for her.

Aggressive Style

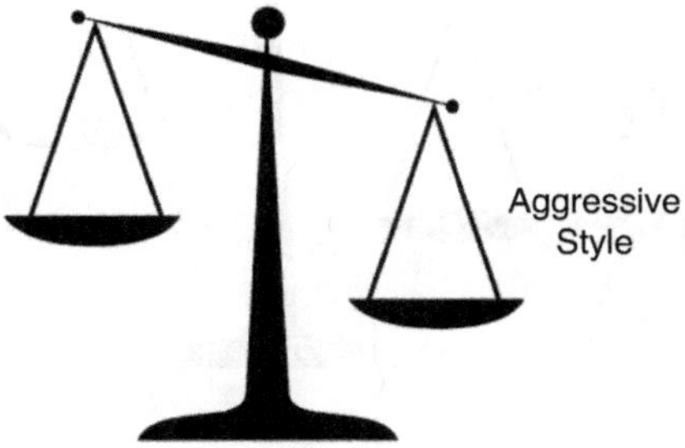

After about 20 minutes, after yelling at her, waving her arms, and hitting her, and even trying to convince herself that it was the best she could do because she is tired of Sofia's disobedience, she begins to remember what happened; the girl's face and her tears begging them to stay a little longer, and the feeling of guilt for what happened begins to surface.

Now let's think about the same scenario, but in this case Sofia's mother communicates in a passive style. When it's time to go home, her mother, anticipating that her daughter will throw a tantrum as soon as she tells her it's time to leave, timidly asks her from the kitchen, "Do you want to go now?" Sofia, after having a great time with her friend, obviously responds with a resounding, "No, I don't want to leave yet!" Her mother, who has already had a difficult day feeling guilty for not spending as much time with Sofia as she would have liked, does not know how to handle the situation without upsetting the girl and, in turn, upsetting herself by confirming her belief that she is a "bad mother" and that her sole and primary goal is to make her daughter happy because life is short.

I know it may seem incredible to you that these things happen, but the truth is that they do. In one of the first workshops I gave on assertive parenting, a mother told me that she no longer knew how to get her son to eat healthy. She was tired of him eating junk foods such as hot dogs and French fries. Just around that time, I had read an example like this in Jane Nelsen's book *Cómo educar con firmeza y cariño (*English title: *Positive Discipline).* A child wanted to eat only French fries and his mother, not knowing what to do to get him to stop eating them, asked Jane how she could change the situation, to which she replied, "Where does he get the French fries?" You can imagine the answer. Well, I took advantage of the fact that I had just read that example and asked the mother with genuine curiosity, "And who buys the chips and sausages for the child?" The mother stared into the distance for about 20 seconds and, nodding her head, replied, "It's true, I'm the one who buys them and brings them home, and not only that, but I also prepare them."

Passive Style

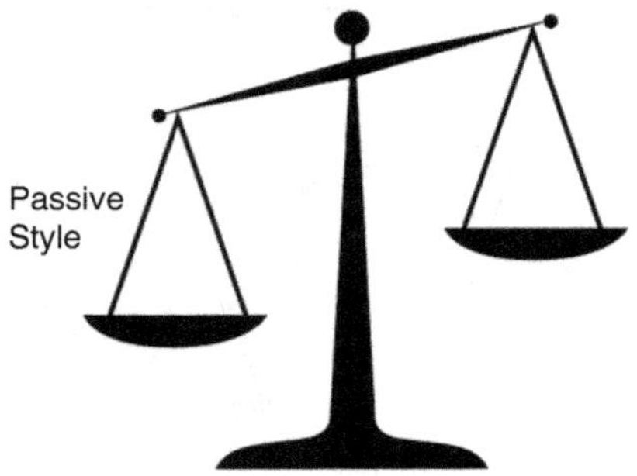

Many people have confused assertive parenting with letting children do whatever they want. Many even refuse to practice assertive parenting because they believe it would be permissive. The truth is that permissiveness or passivity, like aggression and authoritarian parenting, negatively affects our children's mental health. Let's remember what Bowlby said about this: "Mental health is the successful management of conflicts." Therefore, we help our children weather their storms, instead of running away from them.

Now, let's continue with the same example, but in the home of a family that practices assertive parenting. It's time to go home; Sofia and her mother have already agreed in advance how long they would stay at Alexa's house, so when the mother sees that it's almost time to leave, she approaches Sofia, gets down to her level, touches her shoulder, and says, looking her in the eyes, "Honey, we have 20 minutes left before we go home. That means that when the long hand on this clock reaches the 5, where I put this sticker, we'll have to leave."

Assertive Style

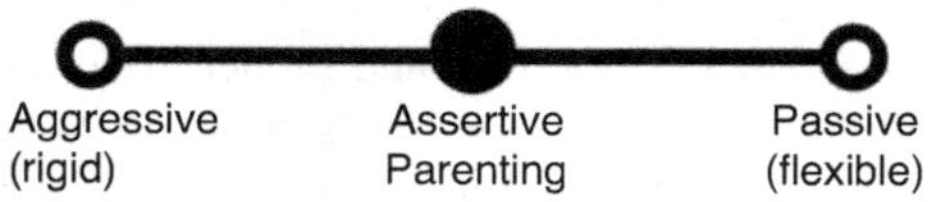

The girl, who is having a great time, gets frustrated and says to her mom:

"I don't want to leave; we can stay a little longer." Her mother, seeing how frustrated her daughter is, replies, "I know you want to spend more time with

Alexa because you love playing with her," but at the same time she responds firmly and affectionately that they can't stay any longer, reminding her of the agreement they had reached and then asking her, "What would you prefer? Do you want me to let you know again when there are 10 minutes left, or do you want to set the hourglass so you can see for yourself? It's up to you." There are several differences here, including before arriving at Alexa's house. Sofia and her mother had already agreed on how long they would stay at her friend's house; this is called anticipation, and it is a key and essential tool in parenting. The next difference is that Sofia's mother makes close eye contact to explain that they have 20 minutes left before leaving. She doesn't tell her that they have to leave at 5 o'clock sharp, nor does she call timidly from the kitchen to ask her if she wants to leave or not. She knows that 20 minutes in a child's mind is nothing. So, she points to the clock to show her when those 20 minutes will be and also involves her in the task. Sofia can decide if she wants to be reminded when there are 10 minutes left before leaving or if she wants to watch the time pass herself with the 20-minute hourglass. Her mother has given her a limited choice, where Sofia can decide within the limits set by her mother.

> Assertive parenting is a way of referring to how we relate to our children with compassion: seeing and treating them as valuable individuals who are capable and worthy of good treatment.

Sofia's mother has performed four important tasks for assertive communication:

> 1 Being able to say no.
> 2 Being able to start, maintain, and end the conversation.
> 3 Being able to validate the other person's emotions or feelings.
> 4 Being able to convey her message firmly, clearly, and kindly.

I combined the word "parenting" with the word "assertiveness," because I deeply believe that our children need our deepest kindness in treating them and, at the same time, our most pleasant firmness in accompanying them, as titled in the wonderful work by Jane Nelsen, creator of the *Positive Discipline*, a book I have mentioned before.

Being assertive parents means being firm when we have to say no to our children, when we set limits, when we are teaching them to be responsible people, and when we encourage their sense of contribution. At the same time, being assertive parents means moving away from shouting, threats, punishments, pinching, slapping, finger pointing, and all those practices that may seem to "work" in the short term because they tend to have the almost immediate effect of eliminating the unwanted behavior we see in our children, but in terms of mental health, they leave us with a high price to pay in the short, medium, and long term.

> When we talk about assertive parenting, we mean parenting with awareness, with intention, and with a roadmap in mind.

In my workshops and counseling sessions, I often tell families that parenting is very similar to driving a car that needs a GPS to reach destination successfully. Our current location represents our present, the place where we are dealing with all those behaviors or situations that challenge us as parents: tantrums, rude answers, fights between siblings, resistance to brushing teeth every morning, complaints, fears, laziness, and everything else that you and I as mothers know all too well. And the destination resembles all those characteristics, skills, and abilities that we want our child to acquire.

> Exercising our motherhood and fatherhood through assertive parenting means educating our children in two ways: first, we educate them for the present, helping them to acquire resources through today's challenges; and second, we educate them for life, so that the skills they have acquired since childhood will be of great use in their adult lives—all with the aim of caring for, cultivating, and protecting their mental health.

No big deal, right?

From my point of view, and especially from the explanatory model with which I have been trained,[6] in order to achieve this goal of educating sufficiently well for the moment and for life, we need to help our children in two ways.

The first is that we provide them with resources that allow them to create a mental framework about themselves as people capable of seeking and asking for help when they need it. The second is that they can create a mental framework about others, fundamentally mom and dad, as people they can turn to and trust when they need help. As we will see in Chapter 5, to develop this belief in our children about themselves as capable individuals, they must first have had someone who believed in them and accompanied them in building an empowering internal dialogue about who they are and what they are capable of achieving. And that designated someone should primarily be their primary attachment figures: their mother and father.

3.2 Myths about assertive parenting

Currently, there are many families who decide to practice conscious parenting that goes beyond meeting physiological needs such as providing food, shelter, or a comfortable bed for their child to sleep peacefully. They have chosen to raise their children by also meeting their emotional, social, and psychological needs. These same families also faced unprecedented amount of information. With advice from psychologists on social media, recommendations from grandmothers who had ten children, parenting lessons from neighbors whose children "turned out well," and admonitions from mothers-in-law who constantly repeat that you still have time to avoid making the same mistakes they did, and all that avalanche of information, most of the time what it does is bring misinformation.

Unfortunately, amid this maelstrom of misinformation, caregivers hear that psychologists are promoting a "crystal generation" in which children around the world can do whatever they want without their parents setting limits. This is, in my opinion, the biggest myth surrounding what we know as assertive parenting, and it has arisen for various reasons:

1 Because there are indeed families who claim to practice assertive parenting when in reality they are passive and permissive parents.
2 Because there are caregivers with an aggressive and authoritarian parenting style whose mental frameworks about themselves and the world around them only allow them to conceive that, in order for a child to learn, they must first feel bad as a way to eliminate any unwanted behavior.
3 Unfortunately, there are parenting professionals who convey the wrong message about what it means to treat a child with respect and dignity. Among other things, these people teach parents to follow the child's own pace in all areas of their life, without setting any assertive limits because this would restrict their freedom. I pause here just to recall what child psychoanalyst Selma Fraiberg said: "The child who is not given limits comes to the conclusion that his parents do not love him." Clear and consistent limits in parenting are a fundamental parameter on which secure attachment is based.

Very often, the relationship between parents and children is affected by a number of invented beliefs that are assumed to be true, and we often accept many of these myths without questioning them. This reminds me of the metaphor of "the deaf frog."[7] If you haven't read it, I think you'll resonate with you, and if you have read it, you'll probably find that it makes more sense now when viewed from the perspective of the myths that surround assertive parenting.

A group of frogs was traveling through the forest when suddenly two of them fell into a deep well. The others gathered around the hole and, when they saw how deep it was, told the fallen frogs that, for all practical purposes, they should consider themselves dead. However, they continued to try to get out of the hole with all their might. The others told them that their efforts would be futile.

Finally, one of the frogs listened to what the others were saying, gave up, and died. The other continued jumping with as much effort as possible. The crowd shouted that it was useless, but the frog kept jumping, with increasing force, until it finally got out of the hole. The others asked, "Didn't you hear what we were saying?" The little frog explained that it was deaf and had thought the others were cheering it on from the edge to try harder and harder to get out of the hole.

How often do we do or say things without knowing why, acting automatically and giving up our parental decisions just because that's how it's always been done? We receive many comments while raising our children. And, like little frogs, some of us may end up giving in and simply doing "for practical purposes" what has always been done, without questioning whether or not it promotes our child's mental health and the development of a secure attachment in their relationship with us. Think about this: your child is unique and your motherhood is unique. Your little one has unique characteristics and requirements that set them apart from other children around them. Not even their siblings are the same!

Most of the time, the best thing we can do is what the "deaf frog" did. Anyone can criticize or express an opinion because we raise our children with their needs in mind; they may call us "soft" or "permissive" for treating them with love and respect. The truth is that we have no control over what people say to us, but we can choose what helps us or not in our work as caregivers.

If the person telling you "don't pick him up when he cries, because he'll get used to being carried" or "let him cry, he'll get tired because they're crocodile tears" is the random woman who sells you bread, then it's easy, you can ignore that person or change the bakery. But if the person who says this to you all the time is your mother-in-law, your brother-in-law, your sister, your father, or any close one, then it hurts and affects you more because you love them and continue to see them, even though you may often wish you could avoid doing so.

If you find yourself in this situation, assertiveness and other actions can be useful in dealing with your family members or close friends when they come to you with their arsenal of myths about respectful parenting.

3.3 What to do when your extended family criticizes your assertive parenting style?

The first and only person who needs to be convinced when you set boundaries for others is yourself. Have you noticed that the more convinced you are about your own boundaries, the more respectful others become of your decisions over time, even if they don't agree with you? It's also true that the more time you spend trying to convince others to respect your boundaries, the more disrespectful they may become toward them. When you try to convince your parents, or anyone else, about your decision to raise your child assertively, that is, with firmness and kindness at the same time, they may perceive your own uncertainty and need for approval, which can send the message, "Do you think what I'm doing is right? I need you to look at me and validate me in order to feel secure." This attitude ultimately causes your boundaries to "fade away" and allows the cycle of seeking approval to continue.

> When you feel like you're about to enter that cycle of seeking approval because others may not agree with your parenting style, take a breath and remind yourself of the following: "My commitment to parenting is to my child. I have my own validation, and that's enough."

Remember that assertive parenting is not limited to being assertive with our children, but also involves being assertive with ourselves and others. This means that you can show empathy and validate that the other person is upset by your parenting style, while also understanding that the emotions or feelings that arise in other people when you set a limit belong to them and not to you. When you set a limit, you are sending the message that you are a different person from the other person, and that you think differently and make different decisions. Ultimately, that is what setting assertive limits is all about.

Let's imagine that your mother gets angry because you don't punish your son when he behaves disruptively; for example, hitting you when he feels frustrated. You have already learned how to deal with this situation using assertive parenting techniques, but your mother thinks it is nonsense and you are a permissive mother. I want to share two ways you could approach this:

1 You can tell them two things that you appreciate about their comment and one thing you don't want them to repeat, while explaining your point of view. Start with something you appreciate, continue with what you don't want them to repeat, and finish with the other action you appreciate. Let's imagine that when this person comes to you, it's because they genuinely care about you and your child and are genuinely concerned about helping you. Thus, what I suggest you say to them might sound like this: "I know you love us very much and that's why you care about the decisions I make (first thing you appreciate). However, I'm not going to do what you say. My partner and I have decided to raise our child this way, and to do so, we are learning how to be the best caregivers we can be in raising our little one, and we are quite committed to it. (Explain your point of view.) I appreciate your concern and love for us." (End with the second action you appreciate.)
2 The second option for addressing this situation is to tell them how you feel. To do this, I recommend using the four steps for nonviolent communication proposed by Marshall Rosenberg:

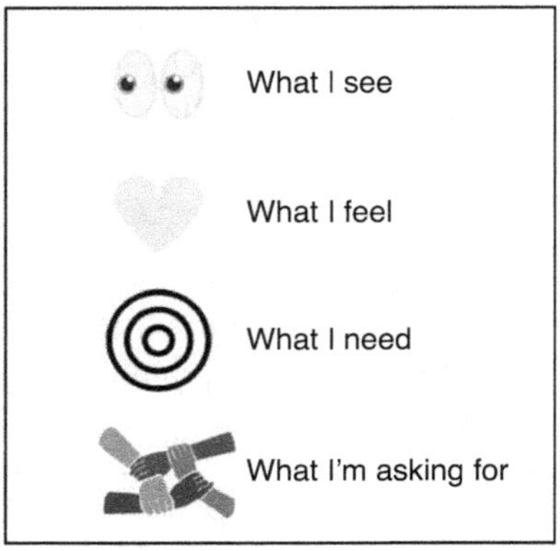

- Observation: Describe what you see, the facts, without making judgments. Act as if you were describing a painting in front of you. When we make judgments, the other person becomes defensive. "You're lazy" carries a judgment. When we describe what we see, there is no judgment: "Mom, this week you've told me twice that I'm a permissive mother because I pick up my son when he cries."
- Feeling: Here you express how you feel about what is happening without insulting or blaming the other person: "Mom, this week you've told me twice that I'm a permissive mother because I pick up my son when he cries. I feel sad when you say that." Instead of: "It makes me sad when you say that."
- Need: Look for the cause of what you are feeling. Perhaps your need is to feel seen. And what you feel is your need, even if it is your mother who causes it. "Mom, this week you've told me twice that I'm a permissive mother because I pick up my son when he cries. It makes me sad when you say that, because I'm very committed to raising my son to the best of my ability with the tools I have."
- Clear request: "I would like us to support and encourage each other. Because I have no doubt how much you love the little one. I know this may be an effort for you, but next time think about it before you say it to me again."

When we practice assertive parenting, it gradually colors the way we see life and relate to others. Conflict is part of our social coexistence and, as such, we will encounter it while raising our children and also in different areas of our lives.

Family life and our social and cultural environment, laden with their own rules, myths, and beliefs that do not favor the way we see and treat our children, teach us to negotiate with these contradictions, and remind us that much of our growth is due precisely to these conflicts. Let us remember that problems are a great opportunity for learning.

3.4 "Bad behavior" is a request for help

Jane Nelsen has a phrase that is widely used in the world of assertive parenting, which had a profound impact on me when I first heard it and continues to have the same effect today: "Where did we get the crazy idea that in order for a child to feel good, we first have to make them feel bad?" I invite you to read it again, thinking about each word, then close your eyes and repeat it.

Perhaps by doing this brief exercise, you will be able to connect more easily with the following anecdote that I experienced at home with my three children.

"Get out of my room! I don't want you in here ever again!" Then she slammed the door. This happened in my house, and that's what I heard one of my daughters say between tears and screams while her younger brother tried to come over to play with her too. As a mom, it hurt me to hear my daughter say that to her brother. However, I knew that joining in the chaos by scolding and punishing her for her behavior was not the best way to understand what was happening and to be able to help her. So I decided to approach her genuinely, as someone who wanted to find out what had happened, and after accompanying her as she gradually calmed down, I asked her with great curiosity, "What happened? I've noticed that this has happened several times over the last week." To which my daughter replied, "Mommy, I don't want Andrés to grab any of the chips and put them in his mouth and swallow them. I don't want anything bad to happen to him because I love him."

My daughter's response reminded me how easy it is to focus on our children's behavior and point fingers at them, even going so far as to label them. When in reality, their behavior is often just a visible reflection of how they feel inside.

When our child hits, pushes, or bites someone, our first thought is usually, "I have to protect the other person," and we may even scold our child for acting the way they did. However, we forget an important detail: at that very moment, our child, even though they may have hurt the other person, also needs protection. And you may ask yourself:

"And how can I protect him?" It can be done by helping him avoid associating his inappropriate behavior with the idea that he is a bad child.

Let's be honest. Parenting—mothering and fathering—is hard; it's difficult. Essentially, it means learning to "lift" our eyes from our own navel so that we can learn to look at and care for a person who is growing up and depends on us. We also know that some moments are more difficult than others. For example, when children scream angrily, when they hit, bite, or push; when they are defiant or rude; or when they refuse to cooperate. It's hard! And it is because, unlike those challenging moments, it is easy to be a conscious mother or father when things are going well, when we read a story together or when we applaud them because they have achieved their goals. On the other hand, when things are not going so well and instead it seems like we are swimming against the tide, practicing assertive parenting becomes more difficult, precisely because we find it hard to be the parents we want to be. Often, we don't know what to do, how to help them, how to effectively teach them so that what happened doesn't happen again. So, what ends up happening is that we also lose control and end up just as frustrated as our children.

> Rudolf Dreikurs said that *discouragement is the root of all bad behavior.* In other words, when a person of any age, and more specifically a child, feels hurt from inside, they act "badly" on the outside.

To understand this, I will draw on the analogy of the iceberg and human behavior proposed by positive discipline.

In workshops with families, I draw an iceberg and then ask parents the following question: What behaviors do you see in your children that currently pose a challenge for you? We write down all the answers on what would be the tip of the iceberg, and they often mention behaviors such as tantrums, lying, aggression, disobedience, or fights between siblings.

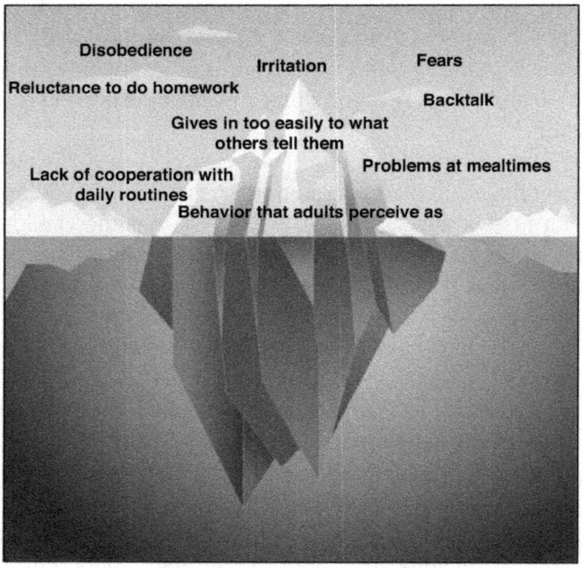

Once we have finished writing down everything that we find challenging about parenting, I ask them: "What would you think if I told you that everything we know as 'bad behavior' is actually a cry for help from your child?" I promise you that there isn't a single workshop where the parents' faces don't light up with a "eureka!" moment, which in Greek means "I've finally figured it out!"

If we start from the premise that our child's behavior is their visible way of communicating something that is not visible to us, we are much more likely to connect with them in that moment and understand that their behavior may be due to a lack of skill, not knowing how to do things differently, not having the linguistic ability to express what is happening to them, or perhaps having a physiological or emotional need that has not been met.

Their behavior may also simply be appropriate for their age. By this I mean, for example, the dreaded tantrums and our insistence on wanting to eliminate them. As we will see when we talk about the brain, these tantrums are often evidence that the child's lower brain (reactive brain) has "hijacked" their upper brain (reflective brain), leaving them completely dysregulated and at its mercy.

If I had focused solely on my daughter's angry face and scream when her brother came over to play with the LEGO, and punished her for talking to him that way, we would have missed the opportunity to learn at least three things. First, my children grow up convinced that when they make a mistake, they have simply made an error, but that does not make them a mistake. Second, when things don't go their way, I will be there to help them deal with their frustration. Third, every conflict is a learning opportunity. In this case, my daughter was able to put into words what she was feeling inside and what prompted her to act that way. And at the same time, when we all calmed down, it was the right moment to teach her how to do things differently next time and to teach her that her words and actions generate a reaction in others. It is our responsibility to use our assertive voice so as not to walk all over others or let them walk all over us. So, in the end, after a brainstorming session that lasted no more than 5 minutes, she and her brother concluded three things:

Next time they would tell him they didn't want to play with him with the LEGO because, being so small, they didn't want him to put the pieces in his mouth and end up swallowing them, which would be bad for everyone. This didn't convince them much because they came to the conclusion that, given his age, he wouldn't understand what they were saying.

Play with the LEGO while he is asleep or lend him another toy that he likes while they continue playing.

The Iceberg Metaphor

The misbehavior you see is your child's misguided solution to a problem you don't see.

Our job is to decipher the code hidden beneath that misbehavior to help our child succeed.

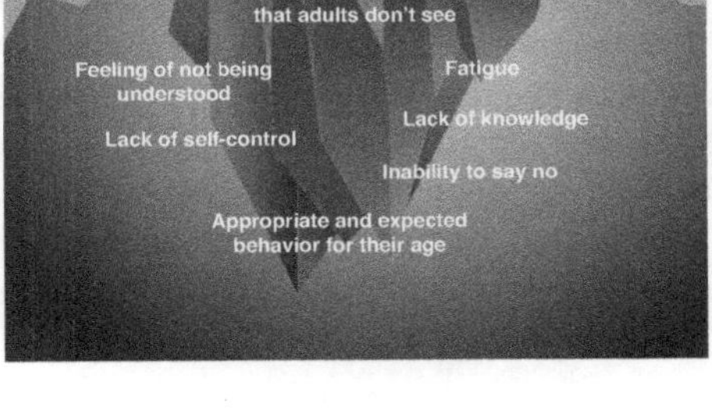

Another point is they should ask me for help if they see that, despite the toy I lent him, he insists on playing with the LEGO.

Moments of conflict are often the most difficult to manage in parenting and in any relationship, yet it is through them that we grow and learn. So the next time a conflict arises—because it will arise even when we have reached agreements—I invite you to put on your detective's suit and your Sherlock Holmes glasses, as Daniel Siegel and Tina Payne Bryson explain in *No-Drama Discipline* (published in Spanish as *Disciplina sin lágrimas*) and with genuine curiosity, set out to look beyond the behavior.

3.4.1 Teaching life skills: five practical points

I want to end this section by sharing some points you should keep in mind when your child exhibits undesirable behavior. This is not a magic wand to change your child's behavior. Instead, it is a way of telling you that sometimes we just need to pause and see our children's behavior for what it is: an SOS, a cry for help.

> Assertive parenting helps you be less reactive and more proactive; in other words, it trains you to anticipate events. You can intuit what might happen before World War III breaks out.

For example, planning to go shopping right after picking up your daughter from school seems like an excellent idea, "since the supermarket is right next to the school, hey, two birds with one stone." And maybe you notice that, when you're fastening your daughter's seatbelt, you brush her arm with yours and she immediately screams, telling you that you've hurt her badly, and starts crying. You can't believe what's happening and just ask yourself, "What did I do now? I barely touched her!" So you scold her and give her the lecture of the year for not appreciating all the effort you've made all morning to finish your work quickly so you can pick her up from school.

You might think that she is perhaps a "very sensitive" child and that lately she cries about everything, or you could see it for what it probably is: an SOS signal. Perhaps you remember that whenever your daughter is tired, she tends to get upset more than your other children or children you know, so maybe next time it would be better to go to the supermarket first to do the shopping and then pick up your daughter from school. Perhaps when you arrive and see her, instead of saying, "Let's hurry up and go shopping," you could say, "I bought the lasagna you told me you wanted so we can have it together for dinner tonight."

It's true that it's not always easy to assume that situation X will trigger situation Y. However, although we can't always predict their behavior, what we can do is anticipate events. This means establishing a nighttime routine together in which they know that at 9 o'clock at night they must be in bed and you will be sitting there with them reading a story.

It also means agreeing in advance on the time your child will return home from their best friend's house, rather than telling them just when it is time to leave. It could also mean humorously interrupting a fight brewing between your children, saying in a funny voice, "Guess what I'm thinking right now?" and responding with a funny, "I don't know either." Or perhaps it could be moving the vase your mother brought you from Morocco, because it looks beautiful on the coffee table, but your children don't yet understand its sentimental value to you. Therefore, assuming our responsibility as adults in everything that can trigger or cause our children's emotional dysregulation, their lack of cooperation, or what we usually call "bad behavior," is something to keep in mind when we intentionally decide to see why our child acts the way they do.

How does this relate to teaching life skills? The following five points are useful reminders, especially when we notice that certain disruptive behaviors recur in our children. The goal is to "look beneath the iceberg" and keep in mind that our job is to teach them the skill they need to learn, rather than punish them for not having developed it yet.

Teaching life skills: five practical points

A → Attribute a positive intention to their 'misbehavior'.

P → Put emphasis on what they should do:

P → Practice the skill your child needs to learn:

L → Lighten their emotional distress with humor and playfulness and help them reconnect.

E → Exercise balance:

Assign a positive intention to their "bad behavior." Don't take it personally; your child does not have the firm intention of making you feel bad. They are learning and need your guidance and direction.

Emphasize what they should do: our children are literal and concrete; they process the information we give them with images rather than words. This is because their left hemisphere, which is responsible for language, is still developing, while their right hemisphere, which is more holistic and nonverbal, specializes in images. So instead of saying, "I've told you a thousand times to brush your teeth and put on your pajamas," try creating a visual routine where they can see the activities that correspond to their nighttime routine. It could be just four images: one showering, one putting on pajamas, one brushing teeth, and one sleeping. To do this, you can print some images of these actions or even print photos of your own child doing each of these activities and make them visible to them during the routine.

Practice the skill you are going to teach and that your child needs to learn; for example, if they find it difficult to ask you for something without shouting, practice this skill in other contexts. For example, practice it through play and make sure that the way you ask them for things is consistent. You cannot ask them to ask without shouting if you shout when you ask them for something. Always remember that anything we want to teach our children, we must first have mastered ourselves.

Use humor and playfulness to lighten their emotional distress and reconnect. Instead of saying, "Stop complaining about everything!" you could try saying something funny and friendly like, "The complaining bug is back, but I wonder how it got in since I made sure to close all the doors and windows. Complaint bug, I've got you! What were you saying, sweetie, that you want an apple? Let's go get it in the kitchen."

Practice balance: If parenting challenges often push you to the extreme of authoritarianism, intentionally set aside time for yourself and self-care. I know this can sometimes be difficult when we can't delegate, but there's something I've learned over my years as a mother: in order to take good care of others, I must first take care of myself. And if authoritarianism has led you to yell even when you're working on improving yourself, practice emphasizing the following to yourself: "I'm a good mother having a hard time. My child is a good child having a hard time. I haven't damaged him forever. I can fix this." And if, on the contrary, you are one of those people who tend to go to extremes of kindness, remember that you have a great advantage, which is your ability to tune into your child's emotional world. Take advantage of these challenges to practice your assertive voice and emphasize the following idea: "I am a good mother having a difficult time. I have not damaged my child by setting a limit. He can handle this, and so can I."

3.5 Understanding the emotional and rational brain to understand child behavior

One mother told me: "My daughter gets frustrated quickly when she loses, no matter what it is: playing Parcheesi, Goose, taking a test, or even a simple riddle. She loses her temper and screams and shouts, and when she was younger she would hit and bite." Another mother said, "With my son, on the other hand, the opposite happens: when he's angry, he doesn't scream, hit, or bite; in fact, he doesn't say anything; it's as if all his anger goes inside. I can tell because his face turns red and he clenches his fists tightly, but he remains motionless."

You might recognize something similar in your children; they might react more like the first mother's child or perhaps like the second mother's, or you might even think, "My child really does get angry," but it does not go either of those two extremes: neither excessive anger nor extreme withdrawal. The truth is that all children in the world become emotionally dysregulated; they get angry, they scream, they feel fear about things that may seem silly to us, and sadness about things that may seem meaningless to us. This may happen with varying frequency, but the truth is that the inability to manage emotions and the inability to remain calm is a fact of childhood. In fact, when a mother tells me, "My two-year-old daughter has tantrums," I am less concerned than when she tells me, "My daughter is two years old and won't even sit down at home." Childhood is a stage in which emotions are close to the surface; children are emotional; their lower brain (brain stem and limbic system), responsible for survival and the emotional world, is predominant, while their upper brain, responsible for logic, order, and executive functions such as empathy and self-control, is still under construction.

I want to explain this to you in the same way that I learned it when I first began to gain a greater understanding of why children behave the way they do and the significant relationship between the behaviors we see in our children and the functioning and maturation of their brains. Therefore, to explain it to you, I must turn once again to Daniel Siegel and Tina Bryson, as, for me, they are two great references on many topics, but specifically on the subject of brain development.

If you pick up any book that contains an image of the brain, you will clearly see how it is divided into two parts. And you probably know that one of these parts is called the "right hemisphere" and the other the "left hemisphere." Else, you may also hear people talk about the "right brain" and the "left brain." This does not mean that we have two brains; these terms simply refer to the brain's two hemispheres: the right and the left. Each part or say each hemisphere, in addition to being separate, performs a different and necessary function, with the shared aim of keeping you, me, our children, and every human being safe and secure.

When the characteristics of the left hemisphere are mentioned, it is usually defined as rational, verbal, temporal, concrete, structured, analytical, decisive, or sequential. Some definitions even highlight how structured it is by referring to it as the "L-hemisphere": linguistic, literal, logical, and linear.

The right hemisphere, on the other hand, is opposite to this, but does not oppose it: it complements it. It is nonverbal, specializing in images, emotions, and autobiographical memories, and is responsible for giving meaning to the experience. It is also responsible for receiving and sending nonverbal signals that facilitate (or hinder) our communication with others; for example, it perceives eye contact, tone of voice, body posture, and gestures; while the left hemisphere is responsible for organizing and putting words to what we experience. It is also worth noting that the right hemisphere is much more closely linked to the "lower" part of the brain, which means that it is more directly influenced by our body. Therefore, it is not surprising to hear that visceral and bodily sensations come from the right hemisphere.

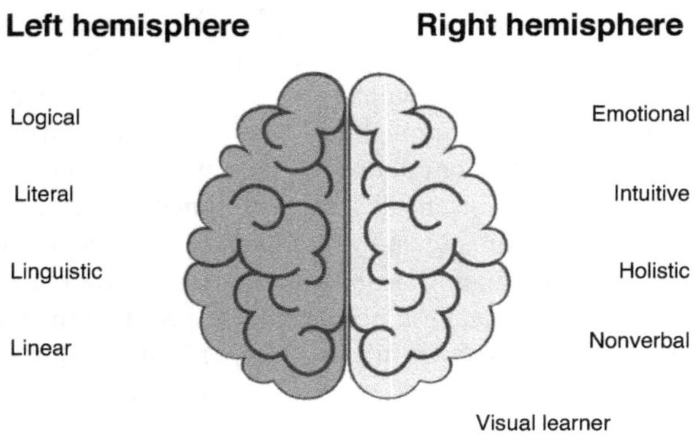

How can knowing this help you in raising your children or supporting your students or patients? Well, science has discovered that the two hemispheres are not only anatomically separate, but also mature differently. And this is precisely where I said:

"Eureka! It all makes sense now. I understand much of my patients' behavior and how to address it," and later, my children's behavior when I became a mother.

To better understand the influence of emotions on behavior, the scientific community maintains that the brain matures in two directions: from bottom to top and from right to left. Rafa Guerrero, a leading figure in the study of the brain and someone I greatly admire, also mentions that the brain develops first from back to front; "the sensory areas (posterior brain) evolve first, followed by the motor areas (anterior brain)."[8]

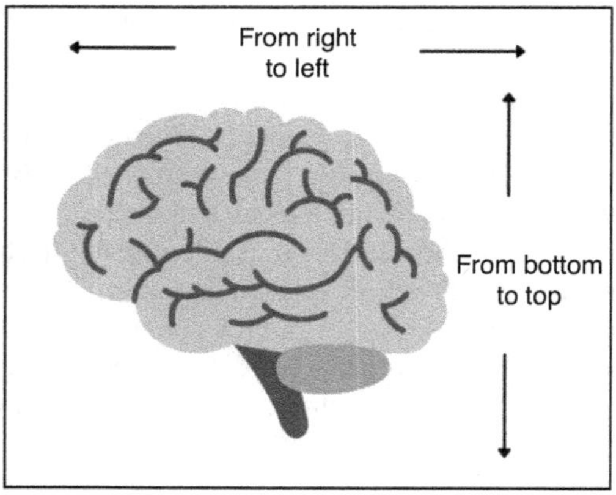

Returning specifically to the maturation of the hemispheres, the points above lead us to the following conclusion.

It is clear that, in young children, especially those who are under 3 years of age, the right hemisphere is predominant. This is because, in terms of maturity, when a child is born, their right hemisphere is much more mature than their left hemisphere. That is why language begins as nonverbal; babies cry when they are hungry, 2-year-olds hit when they want a toy, they do not use the logic and reasoning of the left hemisphere to stop and say: "This car belongs to Samuel and I took it from him to play with. I should have asked him to borrow it instead of snatching it from his hands." It is impossible for a young child to have this left-brain reasoning ability. Their brain is not mature enough for that; they do not have the words or the logical capacity to reach that conclusion. They do not need a "firm hand" to learn to respect other people's things. What this child needs is for her caregiver to "lend" her their reasoning, words, and logic, so that caregiver can (1) approach her with love, compassion, and empathy, understanding that she is a child and is doing the best she can with the tools she has; and (2) invest time in teaching her the skill she needs to learn. Their goal should not be to eliminate the child's behavior. Their goal should be to teach her the skill so that next time she can do it differently.

Knowing that children's right hemisphere, also known as the "emotional brain," predominates gives us greater perspective for understanding why, when they want something, they want it right now, at this very moment. Remember that temporality is the characteristic of the left hemisphere. Children live in the present, here and now; they do not yet have a concept of time. This is a skill they acquire, literally, over time. For this reason, children need anticipation, modeling, clear and concrete instructions, and step-by-step explanations of what they should do (in sequence). In short, we must "exercise" the left hemisphere.

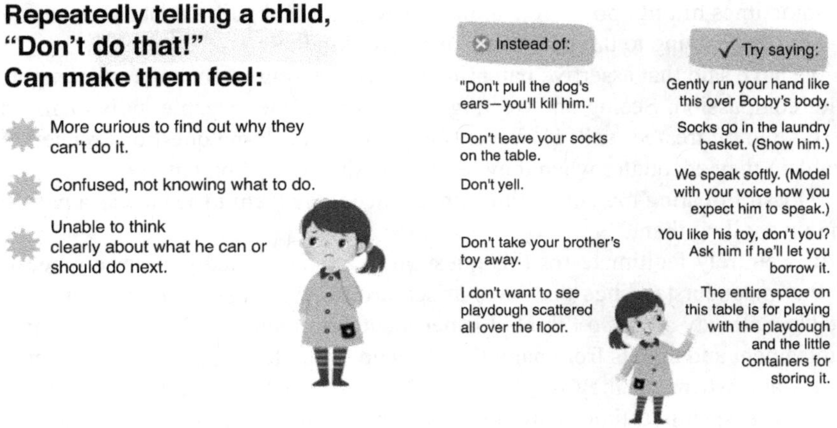
Repeatedly telling a child, "Don't do that!" Can make them feel:
More curious to find out why they can't do it.
Confused, not knowing what to do.
Unable to think clearly about what he can or should do next.
Instead of:
Try saying:
"Don't pull the dog's ears—you'll kill him."
Gently run your hand like this over Bobby's body.
Don't leave your socks on the table.
Socks go in the laundry basket. (Show him.)
Don't yell.
We speak softly. (Model with your voice how you expect him to speak.)
Don't take your brother's toy away.
You like his toy, don't you? Ask him if he'll let you borrow it.
I don't want to see playdough scattered all over the floor.
The entire space on this table is for playing with the playdough and the little containers for storing it.

Our job, then, is not to ensure that logic and reasoning from the right hemisphere predominate in our children, especially in those moments when their emotions overwhelm them; but neither does it consist of leaving them at the mercy of their emotions in order to honor them and give them the recognition they deserve. Doing only the former would leave us with an explanation lacking in meaning and emotional significance, and doing only the latter would leave us trapped in the internal chaos of an intensely lived experience. Therefore, our job is to help our children integrate their two hemispheres (horizontal integration).

Let us recall Bowlby's definition of mental health mentioned earlier: "Mental health involves the satisfactory management of conflicts, the universal conflict being to experience a desire and its opposite simultaneously," and the importance of being firm and kind at the same time in our relationship with our children while we do this. When we help our children integrate their left side with their right, we are giving them the possibility of satisfactorily resolving the chaos that could be caused by experiencing a defensive emotion such as anger or fear (right hemisphere), through the logic, coherence, and order provided by their left hemisphere.

3.6 Raising children "without spoiling them"?

Throughout the day, many of us wake up with the firm intention of practicing discipline that encourages our children, or at least raising them in a way that does not harm them. However, as the challenges of the daily routine arise that same morning, some parents, in order to avoid starting the day with shouting and power struggles, may lean to one side of the scale and go to the extreme of passivity and excessive kindness. However, being pressed for time, the obligation to stick to a schedule and specific tasks, and a lack of cooperation from your children can also be a trigger that causes you to swing abruptly to the other side of the scale: authoritarianism and excessive firmness. Its opposite can also happen. That is, when faced with the first challenge, you may react with excessive firmness, perhaps shouting or sometimes hitting; possibly 5 minutes later, you feel guilty about your reaction and abruptly swing to the other side: excessive kindness.

We have said that assertive parenting means referring to our sons and daughters with compassion. Seeing and treating them as valuable, capable individuals who deserve to be treated well. However, families often ask me questions related to a problem they encounter when they hear about this type of parenting:

"Doesn't treating my child with respect encourage them to see me as a peer and end up spoiling them?"

It is entirely legitimate for this question to arise repeatedly, precisely because of the misunderstandings that have arisen around what assertive parenting is, as we have already seen. So I think it is pertinent to reiterate the fact that eliminating punishment and threats from parenting does not mean letting the child do whatever they want, whenever they want. We need to be clear that "spoiling" has nothing to do with spending time with your children, giving them your undivided attention, accompanying them with compassion when they are upset because things are not going as they expected, reassuring them when they are afraid, picking them up, hugging them, or kissing them. That does not make you "permissive"; rather, it shows that you are your child's life coach and possibly the adult you yourself needed when you were their age.

Remember when child development experts said that if your child had a tantrum, you should send them to the thinking corner to reflect on their bad behavior? The rule was that the amount of time they had to spend in that "thinking corner or chair" should correspond to their age. In other words, if your child is 5 years old, they should sit there for 5 minutes while you ignore them.

I want to emphasize that responding to your child's emotional needs and meeting them well is never synonymous with "spoiling" them. In fact, this is what all caregivers should do in order to nurture the relationship with our children, providing them with a model of themselves as people capable of asking for help when they need it because they are confident that there is someone capable of providing it when they ask for it. And that someone should primarily be their parents. This mental model is the main foundation for promoting our children's emotional well-being, which gives them the assurance that their needs will be met.

However, spoiling does have to do with satisfying our children's desires. Keep in mind that meeting their needs is not the same as responding to their desires. A child may want to eat ice cream right before dinner. Their desire is legitimate, of course, but we cannot turn it into a need. In this case, they may have an unmet physical need (the child hasn't eaten dinner and is hungry). That child needs an adult who empathizes with his desire, but who is also assertive enough to say no, because it's time for dinner. Take a closer look: caregiver is responding to their child's need, but they are not submitting to their desire. If this adult remains consistent in the boundary they have set, and in the subsequent boundaries they will set in other contexts and moments of the child's developmental evolution, that little one will grow up knowing that they will get what they need, even if they don't always get what they want.

And what do we do with the crying that follows that "no"? Accompany them, support them, put it into words, and be compassionate; in other words, meet their needs again. Tuning in to the emotional discomfort caused by the limits we set for our children and responding assertively to their frustration with our unconditional presence has to do with meeting their needs, not giving them what they want. This might sound like this: "You're crying because you want ice cream and I said no. I understand, sweetie; it's hard when things don't go the way we want them to. Tomorrow we can have it for dessert after lunch. You can do this."

> What I am saying is that you have a duty to set boundaries while raising your children. Above all, boundaries that have to do with their own safety, health, and respect. And, at the same time, your child has the right to feel frustrated when you set them.

Assertive parenting is about accompanying our children as they weather the storm, not rescuing them to get them out of it. We want our children to grow up feeling capable, useful, cared for, seen, and connected to their secure base. By doing this, we are fostering their autonomy because the way to get our children to transition from dependence to autonomy is by feeling connected, secure, and in tune with us. In doing so, we are fulfilling the dual goal of assertive parenting: educating them for the moment and for life.

At this point, and to conclude, it is important to be clear about exactly what needs a caregiver should be aware of and meet in order to answer the question: "How do I know if I am meeting an emotional need and not constantly satisfying my child's desire?" Let's remember that desires will always be legitimate: desiring is human, it is part of being alive; we validate desires, but constantly satisfying our children's desires can be counterproductive. We validate their desires, but we meet their needs.

3.6.1 The 15 basic needs every caregiver should know for assertive parenting

The following is the list of 15 emotional needs that are based on what I learned during my training in brief psychotherapy with children and adolescents at the Spanish Society of Psychosomatic Medicine and Psychotherapy:

1. Explicit love: gaze, words, contact.
2. Emotional regulation: recognition, labeling, legitimization, regulation, expression.
3. Time with complete attention.
4. Safety/protection.
5. Emotional attunement: feeling heard, understood, seen.
6. Mobilization/response: the opposite is emotional neglect.
7. Appropriate role deployment: the task of caring is the adult's; the child is not responsible for the adult's emotional world.
8. Clear boundaries.
9. Appreciation, acceptance, respect.
10. Sufficient and appropriate stimulation/motivation.
11. Resources/autonomy.
12. Sense of belonging.
13. Reflective capacity/mentalization.
14. Identity.
15. Magic: unconditional love is the most powerful "magic" that exists to accompany a child in their development process.

Notes

1. Barudy, J., and Dantagnan, M. (2013). *Los buenos tratos a la infancia. Parentalidad, apego y resiliencia.*. Barcelona: Gedisa.
2. Bowlby, J. (1989). *Una base segura: aplicaciones clínicas de la teoría del apego*. Barcelona: Paidós Ibérica.
3. Convention on the Rights of the Child. The Convention on the Rights of the Child (CRC) is an international treaty that recognizes the human rights of children, defined as persons under the age of 18, and obliges governments to comply with them, as well as other agents such as parents, health professionals, and teachers. (*Source*: www.unicef.es.)

4 Dreikurs, R. (1991). *Children: The Challenge: The Classic Work on Improving Parent-Child Relations: Intelligent, Humane, and Eminently Practical*. Plume.
5 Siegel, D., and Bryson, T.P. (2012). *El cerebro del niño. 12 estrategias revolucionarias para cultivar la mente en desarrollo de tu hijo*. Barcelona: Alba.
6 I have adopted my training model from Begoña Aznárez and José Luis Marín, presidents of the Spanish Society of Psychosomatic Medicine and Psychotherapy, and it is based on attachment theory, trauma theory, and family systems theory.
7 Bernal, M., and Lopera, J. (2002). *La culpa es de la vaca. Anécdotas, parábolas, fábulas y reflexiones sobre el liderazgo*. Bogotá: Intermedio Editores Ltda.
8 Guerrero, R. (2020b). *Educar en el vínculo*. Barcelona: Plataforma Actual.

Chapter 4

The child and the gaze of their caregivers

> The gaze of another is vital because it shapes our future life: Am I desirable?
> (Boris Cyrulnik)

Let's begin this chapter by trying to remember how our parents or other significant adults, who somehow also shaped our childhood, looked at us.

How did they look at you when you made a mistake? How did they look at you when you got something right? How did they look at you when they asked you something and you didn't have an answer? Was it an unconditional or judgmental look? Was it a look that made you feel secure or, on the contrary, made you feel ashamed, afraid, angry, or guilty?

I learned from my teacher, Begoña Aznárez, that the gaze sustains the bond, that a compassionate gaze generates the trust that goes beyond knowing that the other person is my caregiver and the one who gave birth to me, and that it is really based on knowing and feeling loved and accepted unconditionally for who we are. The gaze of others, especially our caregivers, is so important that it can lift us up and help us overcome obstacles, or sink us into the deepest guilt. Therefore, the guideline to keep in mind is being intentional when we look at our children while raising them. When I say intentional, I mean being aware of the gaze we choose to cast on our children, both when they get it right and when they get it wrong, bearing in mind that this will determine how they will see themselves in future.

Eric Berne, creator of transactional analysis, spoke of the "life script"[1] as the narrative that each person has internalized about themselves and the world around them. And how this script is fundamentally influenced by the mandates, views, and roles that each person has received in their immediate environment, that is, fundamentally in their family nucleus, while interacting with their caregivers, especially in those early years of life when human beings are so dependent and at the same time so in need of clinging to a vital figure as a means of survival.

> Eric Berne drew on to fairy tales to say that we are all born princes or princesses until our parents' gaze turns us into toads or frogs.

DOI: 10.4324/9781003784487-4

It depends largely on the view we have received from those we care about, whether the script we have internalized about ourselves is more like that of princes or princesses or toads or frogs.

If we take the time to think about what we say to ourselves, especially when we make mistakes, we may be surprised to find that the internal language we use with ourselves is very similar to the language used with us in our childhood. A young child begins to construct their idea of themselves based on the idea that their caregivers first formed about them. The words used with us in childhood shape the way we learn to see ourselves, just as the words we use with our children can become the mirror in which they learn to see themselves. Hence, the importance of being intentional.

This time, I turn to Stephen Karpman and his well-known model of the "Karpman drama triangle" to explore further the importance of our gaze in the construction of our children's identity and how, in turn, the gaze of our caregivers has influenced our own identity and way of relating to others.

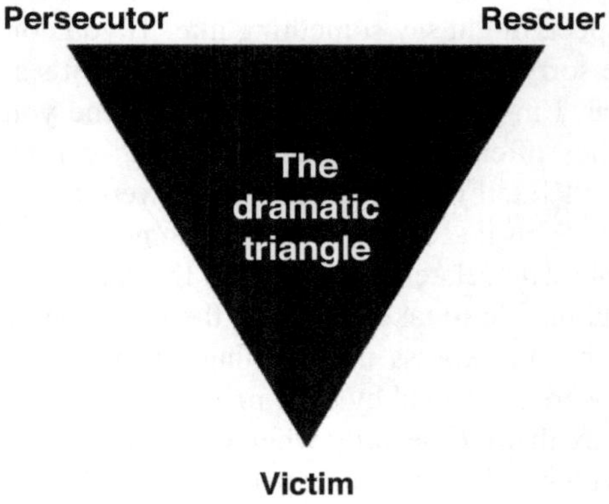

Karpman's drama triangle is a model often used in psychotherapy to understand conflicts and their dynamics within interpersonal relationships. This model views conflicts as the product of internal psychological processes within each person that lead them to unconsciously adopt *conflicting roles* in order to survive. These roles are: victim, persecutor, and rescuer. This author starts from the premise that all dysfunctional relationships revolve around the drama triangle[2] and that each "protagonist of the drama" starts from one of three important roles: rescuer, victim, or persecutor in relation to the other "actor," who is usually the antagonist, who also has their own role within the triangle. In other words, when you have a conflict with another person, whether it be your child, partner, father-in-law, sister-in-law, brother, or aunt, and, as a result, you feel hurt, sad, angry, ashamed, guilty, despised, humiliated, fearful, anxious, etc., you are unconsciously placing yourself at one of the vertices of the triangle and, at the same time, placing the others at the other vertices. These roles are not static; you can switch from one to another at different times. For example, when there is a change in a specific situation, the people involved often move within the triangle, changing roles; the "persecutor" may become the "victim" and the "rescuer" may end up becoming the "persecutor." In other words, the roles are not fixed, but the same person can take on one role or another, depending on the situation or the moment they are in.

One might assume that, in order to be inside the triangle, there would need to be conflictual interaction between three or more people. However, if there is conflict between two people, they could also be located within the drama triangle since, within it, all the "actors," although they act from their own role, start from the basis that they are "victims," which makes the relationship more tense and stressful.

How can we observe this within the context of parenting, and how does it relate to the gaze and emotional bond between parents and children? To answer this question, we will first describe the characteristics of each role, focusing specifically on parenting, and then illustrate them with an example.

"Persecutor" role: The persecutor role occurs when the caregiver cares about their children but at the same time blames, shames, or reproaches them when they do not change or behave as desired. A caregiver in this role, when their child does not do what they expect, might say something like "If you don't do what I tell you right now, you'll be sorry." Or "I don't understand why it's so hard for you to do everything I tell you. I'm your mother and you owe me your life! Never forget that!" In addition, they often seek support for their speech from third parties, for example, "Tomorrow I'll tell your teacher that you were lazy all day and didn't do your homework." Or "You'll see when Dad gets home and I tell him."

Deep down, people who relate to others from the role of followers feel uneasy, insecure, fragile, and unable to take charge of their own emotions. Many of them learned as children not to express their feelings in order to protect themselves, either because they were neglected by their primary attachment figures or because they were punished by them, especially when emotions such as anger or fear were expressed. Feeling vulnerable can be an experience that they perceive as dangerous.

In her discussion of Karpman's drama triangle, Gill Edwards states: "It is not uncommon for persecutors to have suffered abuse (emotional, physical, or sexual) in their childhood, and who, as a result, have learned to survive by identifying with the figure (or figures) of a critical parent prone to manipulating, shaming, or controlling others. This defense mechanism is known as "identification with the aggressor" and provides them with a resistant outer shell".

When a caregiver assumes the role of persecutor, it can generate fear, shame, and/or guilt in their children. This is probably because their behavior is driven by the amount of pent-up anger that they have not had the opportunity to validate, name, embrace, cry about, or process with the support of that significant other who should have been their secure base. As a result, their anger often comes out explosively, hurting those around them, who are usually part of their inner circle.

"Rescuer" role: It is also known as "responsible parent." When caregivers identify with this role, they tend to show great concern for meeting not only the needs of their children and partner, but also their desires, even if this means neglecting their own needs. Caregivers who operate in this role often do things they don't want to do, but because they have a low tolerance for conflict, they do everything in their power to keep the peace, even if doing so leaves them feeling internally conflicted. This role is known as the "rescuer" because the parent who assumes this role tries to help their child in ways that are often neither healthy nor empowering. Colloquially, we refer to these parents as "overprotective" because, instead of empowering their children for life, they disable them by doing for them what they would be capable of doing for themselves. This caregiver's discourse might sound something like "Don't worry about anything, I'm here to do it for you."

Gill Edwards says that rescuers have become accustomed to taking an interest in matters outside the realm of their own needs and to being guided by what those around them want. They think obsessively about others and their problems, and although their behavior has the virtue of great empathy, their lives are subject to the agendas of others. Everyone else matters more to them than themselves. Helping and caring for others becomes an addiction; for the rescuer, it is as if life passes them by without touching them. Their feelings and needs have become so secondary that they even have difficulty recognizing what they really feel or want.[3]

This attitude may be due to the fact that they only feel truly seen and valued when they do something for others. This behavior often stems from families who openly praise their children when they show solidarity or interest in others but punish and reprimand the child when they do not want to share, for example, their new toy or refuse to lend their ball to their cousin who has come to visit. Therefore, it is not surprising that a caregiver who assumes this role has become accustomed to constantly seeking the approval of others by being kind and overly helpful, even if this means denying and invalidating their own needs and emotions.

"Victim" role: This role is usually assumed under the influence of the persecutor or rescuer, so the person's inner dialogue tends to be along the lines of "poor me." In this role, the person usually sees themselves as a victim of circumstances, of their family, of the system, or of life itself, and often displays an attitude of helplessness and inability to deal with their own discomfort or with what is troubling them. When you act in this role, you may come across as a weak, misunderstood person, and you may even manipulate others in order to receive the care and protection you so desire. When a caregiver constantly plays this role in their relationship with their child, they may send a nonverbal message to their child saying, "Poor me, I've done so much for you, and this is how you behave."

Now let's look at all of this with an example:

Six-year-old daughter says, "I'm not going to eat cereal for breakfast. I've told you a thousand times that I don't like it."

Father assumes the role of persecutor (addressing his daughter): "You eat everything, period. You're not in charge in this house."

Mother assumes the role of rescuer (addressing the father): "Don't talk to her like that. Let's not start the morning this way. It's no trouble for me to make her something different."

Six-year-old daughter assumes the role of victim (starts crying): "That's why I love Mom more than you, because you never listen to me."

Mother, now assuming the role of persecutor (addressing the father): "Do you realize how much fear you instill in others? You're very rigid."

Father: "Come on, man! Now it turns out that I'm the one who started all this."

As I said at the beginning, roles are not fixed; the same person can take on one role or another, depending on the situation or the moment. We see that the mother has moved from the role of "rescuer" of the daughter to the role of "persecutor" of the father.

Our parenting style, family rules, and the parenting patterns that we bring from our own childhood can lead us to unconsciously adopt conflicting basic roles and, in turn, "assign" other roles to our children as we interact with them. This creates friction in the bond between the child and their caregiver, generating greater conflict and dysfunction in the relationship. One of the first things we can do to transform this situation is to choose to be aware of the place from which we are operating most of the time when interacting with our children and the family system in general. The idea is not to label ourselves as "I am a persecutor, victim, or rescuer," but to observe how our own decisions and behavior on a daily basis may in turn be influencing our children's behavior, so that we can move on to a second step, which consists of being intentional when interacting with them. In other words, we need to get out of the autopilot mode that pushes us to react and choose to work on ourselves to learn to respond with greater awareness. We need to understand that, as we move toward this new level, we will make many mistakes, and that it is precisely these mistakes that will give us opportunities to continue learning. We will discuss all of this in the next section.

4.1 From persecutors, rescuers, or victims to guardians of resilience

"How do you see me?" This is one of the questions that arises in children as they grow up. They will start by asking themselves how their parents see them, then how their teacher sees them, and then how their friends see them. There is a lot of content in that question.

> Do you remember when, as a child, a single glance from your parents communicated what they expected of you? And also how you would flee from the gaze of strangers, possibly hiding between your caregivers' legs or perhaps covering your eyes.

It seemed that everything ended there: "If I don't look at them, it's as if they no longer exist in my world." However, as we grew up and interacted with the people who mattered most to us, that gaze became engraved in our hearts. Above all, the gaze of our key figures, who are usually dad and/or mom, but who could also have been a grandmother, uncle, stepmother, or the person(s) who took care of us during our early years.

As we have seen, children construct an idea about themselves mainly through the eyes of their primary caregivers. As Siegel and Bryson (2020) say, children learn who they are and who they can and should be, both in good times and bad, through their interactions with us, their parents.[4]

The parenting style we exercise as parents and the way we relate to and treat our children can lead them to adopt one role or another in their interaction with us. Sometimes, when there is friction in the relationship, the role of each member can be framed within one of the basic conflicting roles of the drama triangle, creating a loop and generating greater disconnection in the parent-child relationship.

4.1.1 What can we do to break the cycle and repair our relationship with our children?

In this regard, I love to refer to the term used by Boris Cyrulnik, "resilience tutors," which I use to suggest that one of the best tasks we can carry out while raising and interacting with our children is to be that guide, that support, and that tutor on whom our child can rely as they grow, make mistakes, and learn.

It is like the stake placed beside a plant to support its growth. We help the plant by placing the stake beside it so that it can grow as well as possible, and we provide it with the care it cannot provide for itself.

Learning to see our child's unique nature leads us to provide them with the care they need, which will help them to be who they are and discover who they are. But let's be honest, it sounds simple, but it's not always easy. However, it's worth all the effort, because your child will learn to see themselves as a capable and loved person fundamentally through the way you treat them.

> In this sense, assertive parenting is the means by which you can learn to become that resilience coach or, as I call it, your child's life coach. But first, stop and think about this: assertive parenting is not the goal, but rather the means by which you train yourself every day to become that resilience coach your child needs and move toward the desired goal, which is to build a secure attachment with your child.

This is what we ultimately want to provide for our children, and it is the most important task we can undertake as parents. Secure attachment increases your children's ability to overcome obstacles, boosts their mental health, and helps them build a much more positive view of themselves and the world around them. It allows them to form quality relationships and increases their likelihood of academic and professional success, as demonstrated by various studies.

Does this mean that there is no room for error in parenting? No. It is too difficult to parent without making mistakes, and not only difficult, but impossible. It's more about your child growing up with the certainty that, even if they make mistakes, they know they can count on you time and time again. As we will see in the chapter on secure attachment, the trust and security that children receive from their parents reduce the levels of stress generated by situations over which they have no control or when things don't go as expected. In other words, an outcome of building secure attachment with your children is that they learn to cope with difficult situations based on the idea that they have the security and confidence that, even if they make mistakes, your love and relationship with them will remain safe. And it is precisely this security and confidence that will allow them to try again based on the assumption: "I am capable, I can do this."

Let's summarize: the primary goal of parenting is to build a secure attachment with our children. We achieve this by relating to them with confidence, security, and an intentional, compassionate, and unconditional gaze that empowers them for life. To this end, assertive parenting is the vehicle that allows us to see the role we are playing in our relationship with them and, at the same time, the parenting style we are using. Thus, understanding that our parenting style and the gaze we have placed on our children have influenced the concept they have built about themselves and others helps us to be more aware of what may be causing conflict in the relationship and what we must do intentionally to become the guardians of resilience that our children need.

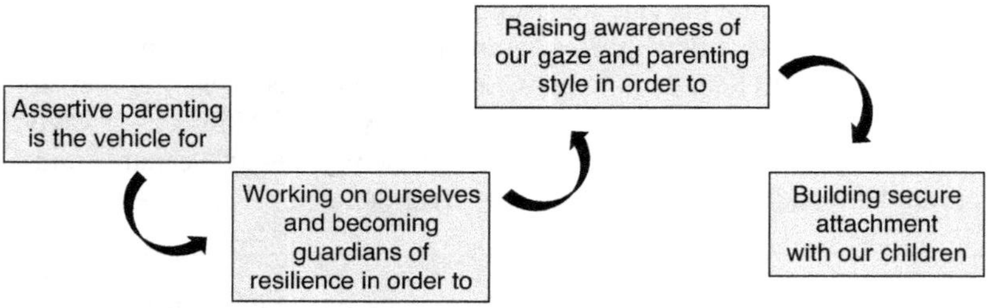

4.2 How does a child build a belief about themselves? And how can we help them?

Based on how those who matter see them and treat them, children form an idea of how they see themselves, how they treat themselves, and how they talk to themselves.

A study conducted by psychologists Robert Rosenthal and Leonore Jacobson in the 1960s, called *the Pygmalion effect*, shows how the expectations and beliefs that adults have about children condition and influence their behavior, abilities, effort, and, ultimately, the concept they build about themselves. It should be noted that this influence is mainly exerted by the adults who are important in the child's life.

This study was conducted with elementary school children. Before the school year began, new teachers at the school were told that a group of students had taken an intelligence test and that 20% of them had achieved outstanding results. They were told that these gifted children would probably be the ones with the best academic results throughout the school year, compared to the other children who had below-average results and who, therefore, were highly likely to perform just as poorly.

Eight months later, the teachers who participated in the experiment were brought together to analyze the results.

The results showed that children labeled at the beginning of the school year as having a high IQ performed well and were highly motivated to learn; their grades were above average. In contrast, the other children labeled as "children with low IQs" performed poorly and were unmotivated to learn.

Not only did they have grades well below average, but teachers also reported that these students were unmotivated and had a low predisposition to learn.

So far, nothing could be surprising. But do you know what really caused astonishment? That no intelligence tests were ever administered, and that there was no specific evidence to show that any of these children were more academically gifted than others. Twenty percent of these children were chosen at random. So, how is it possible that this happened and that, in fact, the students who were said to have better intellectual performance achieved better academic results, while those who were said to have less intellectual advantage achieved poorer academic performance at the end of the course?

The answer lies in what is known as *the Pygmalion effect.* Children who were said to have an academic advantage were treated as such, which led them to believe it and act accordingly. Similarly, children who were identified as having low IQs were treated as such, which also led them to believe it and act accordingly.

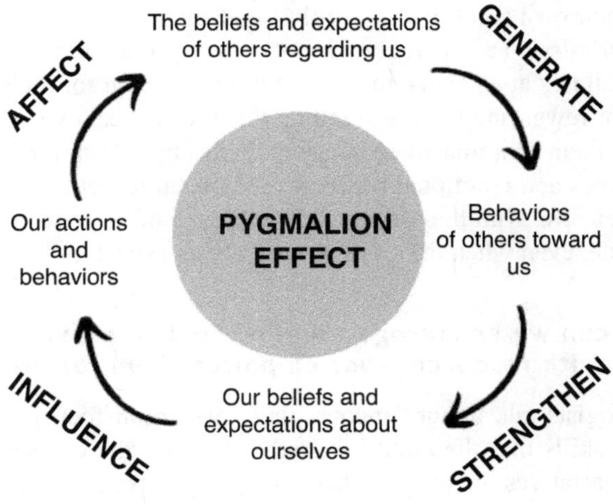

Generally, when an adult interacts with a child, whether it is their own child or a student, based on the idea that the child has the ability to perform specific tasks appropriate for their age, their expectations are sufficient to make them try harder to help the child learn, as they trust in the child's abilities and are confident that the child can give more of themselves by facilitating their learning when they encounter obstacles. The opposite is also true. When an adult does not expect much from a child, whether academically, emotionally, or behaviorally, that same adult often makes very little effort to help the child learn the skills they need. And when that child has a difficulty, the adult often has a preconceived notion about the child's emotional or cognitive abilities, which might sound something like "it's impossible," "they won't be able to do it," "they aren't capable," or "I've done everything I can and nothing has changed," and the child acts in accordance with this preconceived idea of the adult, since that is how they are treated both verbally and non-verbally.

Psychologist Martin Seligman calls the internal discourse that children create about themselves and the world around them *an explanatory style.* He also says that children's pessimism is partly learned from the adults they respect and spend most of their time with: parents, teachers, and coaches. Our children are like sponges: they absorb both what we say and how we say it.[5]

When children perceive their reality through all their senses, a series of reactions, known as *internal experience*, are generated within them. This, in turn, generates a response that manifests itself through thoughts, emotions, bodily sensations, and actions. These four elements, common to all experiences, lead children to interpret what they have experienced, based on how their caregivers attuned themselves to their inner experience and responded to it. From there, based on the absence or presence of appropriate parental support or lack thereof, children construct a belief about themselves and others and act accordingly.

Given what we have seen, we might ask ourselves what we can do to help our children build an image and belief about themselves that are as realistic as possible in relation to their own emotional, cognitive, and social resources.

You see, your mission as a caregiver is not to avoid your child from experiencing mistakes and failures at all costs, to constantly praise them for their achievements and victories, or rewarding them and telling them how great everything they do is in order to give them an immaculate image of themselves. Your job is to equip them with the resources and emotional resilience they need to get through the difficult moments in their life, with the assurance that in each of those moments they have the skills to cope, even when things don't turn out as expected.

4.2.1 How can we encourage them while also providing them with resources that empower them for life?

When psychologists talk about "encouraging," we mean focusing on the effort, resources, and skills that the child has, rather than on the expectations, desires, judgments, or narratives of approval that adults may make or say about the child's performance.

> Telling a child "very good" does not help them build a belief about themselves as someone capable. However, it will always be much better to say "very good" than to criticize, judge, or threaten them when they make a mistake. I have no doubt about that.

The problem with overusing phrases such as "very good," "you did it just as I expected," or "I'm so happy you did it the way I told you" when our child has achieved something or said something that makes us happy as parents is that, with such praise, we are teaching them to base their self-worth on the approval and the judgment of others. We motivate them to continue painting, helping, singing, or doing whatever it takes to get that "very good," that is, we are motivating their behavior through the approval or disapproval they may get from others.

At the behavioral level, what we have mentioned occurs, that is, children feel the need to get the attention of those who matter to them through the approval of their actions. At the cerebral level, what we are doing is activating their brain's pleasure circuit, also called the "mesocorticolimbic circuit," which, by releasing dopamine, creates the need to seek this external approval in the child again in order to hear once more what made them feel valuable.

When children are young, they expect this from us; when they grow up, they will expect it from others. Their internal dialogue and the belief they build about their worth may sound something like "If I do this and they tell me it's okay, then I am valuable. If they don't say anything or don't like it, then I am not valuable."

The proposal, as suggested by positive discipline, is to learn to "encourage" rather than "praise." *Encouragement* helps children feel valuable without depending exclusively on the approval of others and without constantly seeking to please them in order to feel seen, heard, and taken into account. When we encourage, we nurture their self-esteem because, instead of labeling them as good or bad, smart or clumsy, we highlight their effort, their process, and their ideas.

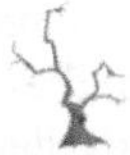

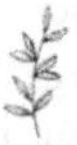

Instead of...	**Try...**
Very good. You did it just as I expected you to.	You worked hard and you did it. I can imagine how satisfied you must feel.
If I hadn't insisted that you finish it, you wouldn't have succeeded.	You made a mistake and kept trying. How do you feel?
I disagree. Just focus on studying, period.	I really value each of your ideas. Which one do you think can help you achieve your goal?

To find out if you are an encouraging or praising caregiver, I invite you to think about the statements you usually use and ask yourself the following:

> Does what I say lead my children to look at their abilities and effort, or to seek only my approval to feel valuable?
>
> Am I encouraging my children to look at their entire learning process or strictly at whether or not he has achieved his goal?
>
> Do my words take my children's point of view into account, or do they focus exclusively on what I consider important?

4.3 I'm ok, you're ok

Eric Berne, whom we discussed in Chapter 3, also proposed, in his theory of transactional analysis, four existential positions from which we relate to each other and see the world:

> I am well, you are well.
> I am well, you are unwell.
> I am unwell, you are well.
> I am unwell, you are unwell.

This existential position would be the way we position ourselves in relation to others and act accordingly:

Who am I? How much value do I have as a person? Who are others and how much value do they have? What is the world around me like?

When raising children, the ideal would be to relate to them from a position of "I'm okay, you're okay." However, in everyday life, this may not be the case, and we may end up in a position of "I'm okay, you're not okay," which is what usually happens when parents consider psychological help to help their child change their behavior. Or "you're okay, I'm not," when our own history makes us feel unable to approach parenting well enough, or, in the worst case, "I'm bad, you're bad," where caregivers feel completely lacking in personal resources and, at the same time, unable to provide the child with the tools and skills they need for life.

Although it is true that in parenting we may meet parents who relate to their children from any of these four existential positions proposed by Eric Berne, I am going to focus exclusively on the one referring to "I'm OK, You're wrong" and how to work to move the relationship with our child from there to one that is more like "I'm okay, you're okay."

There is nothing more encouraging for a child than feeling seen, important, accepted, and secure in the love of their parents. Children are small, dependent, and egocentric, and recreate themselves in the world of fantasy. Just as they can come to believe that a man is capable of entering their home through the chimney to leave them gifts at Christmas, or that three kings arrive every January 6 to brighten their mornings, that same little one can contemplate the idea that their parents may stop loving them when they make a mistake or when they behave in a way that is not what their parents expect. This is precisely because in childhood, due to their egocentric bias, "the child's world is small" and they may conceive that everything good and unpleasant that happens to them is due to what they do, say, or think.

Positive discipline maintains that all behavior is our child's way of communicating how their inner world is, and that the beliefs children form about themselves and others are colored precisely by their difficulty in interpreting the world beyond their egocentric thinking. In fact, one of Rudolf Dreikurs' most frequently quoted statements in workshops taught by trainers who follow this approach is that children are very good at perceiving, but very poor at interpreting. In other words, it doesn't matter how much we know we love our children; what matters is knowing how they are interpreting the love we feel for them, because it is precisely through that interpretation that the belief motivating their behavior is generated.

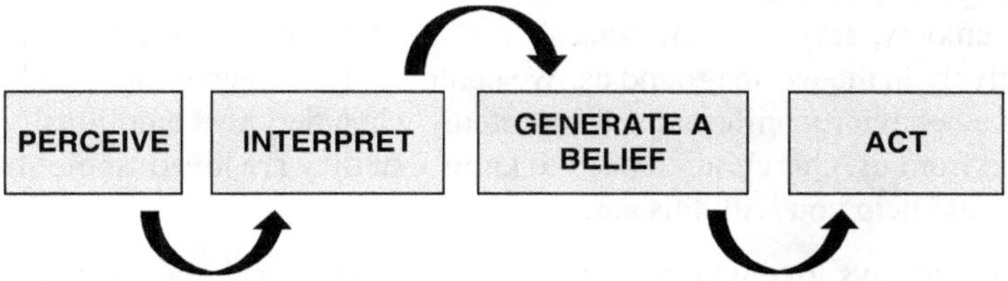

Four-year-old Sofia has become a big sister; her daily routine of going to the park, playing, showering, and reading stories at night has changed with the birth of her new baby brother. Sofia now watches her parents talk lovingly to someone who is completely new to her. She observes that almost overnight, her mother carries this "stranger" in her arms all the time; even when she wakes up at night, she sees her mother with the baby in her arms, changing his diaper, or feeding him. Her parents report that Sofia has now started to wet and soil herself, even though she had already outgrown this stage. They also say that she seems more irritable and that the school has told them she has started hitting and biting her classmates. Sofia's parents say they don't understand what is happening and don't believe it is jealousy because they see the girl being very affectionate with her little brother and very proud to say she is a big sister.

This example often illustrates how our children form beliefs and act accordingly. Sofia has noticed that her world has changed overnight, her routines are different, and her parents are no longer there for her 24 hours a day. What's more, she sees them devoted day and night to someone else. Now she has to share her time with a new family member. At 4 years old, with an egocentric mindset that attributes everything that happens around her to herself, Sofia has interpreted the change in her routine and everything that it entails as a "threat" to her parents' love for her. Let's remember that a child's greatest fear is believing that mom or dad might stop loving them. Is it true that Sofia's parents' love has diminished or is about to change because of the birth of their new child? Of course not, but this example illustrates that it doesn't matter how much love we know we feel for our children, what is important is to understand how they are interpreting the love we feel for them in their inner world. Understanding how they feel and how they perceive the world around them helps us understand much of their behavior.

This is the first step in moving from "I'm right, you're wrong" to "I'm right, you're right."

When we understand that behavior is largely a form of communication, we can look beyond the behavior itself.

If we view our child's behavior as a "megaphone" that communicates their inner state, then it will be easier to see their behavior as a cry for help, rather than a personal attack or a tool our child uses to "get their way."

What you can do:

1 Reassure them by expressing your love explicitly: Stephen Porges, author of the polyvagal theory and whom we will mention again when we talk about childhood anxiety, says that returning to a state of security is the basis for acting adaptively in the world around us. We could say that much of our children's disruptive behavior manifests itself repeatedly when they feel emotionally disconnected from us. Our children need to know that they are loved; some statements that could help you with this are:

   - I will always love you: whether you are happy or sad, angry or calm, afraid or determined.
   - I'll be here for you for as long as it takes.
   - Would you like me to give you a hug?
   - There's no rush. We can talk whenever you want.
   - Would you like to talk about how you feel?
   - Even though we sometimes feel uncomfortable in our bodies, it's normal to feel anger, fear, or sadness.
   - I'm here for you, sweetheart.
   - Sometimes you don't have to say anything: just listening without judgment is enough.

2 Empathize with their emotions without justifying their behavior. When you do this, you are tuning into their inner world and, as Daniel Siegel says, "your child feels felt." When you understand that expressing anger, fear, or sadness is not bad behavior but a reaction to a stimulus perceived as threatening to your child, you can begin to see them more compassionately. This does not mean that you justify all kinds of behavior, especially when it hurts others. What it means is that you understand why they are acting the way they are and where they are coming from. One way that can help you with this point is to refer to a moment in your life, preferably from your childhood, when you experienced the same or something similar to what they are experiencing.

3 Redirect their behavior by assertively sharing what you think. To do this, it will be essential that you first tune in to their emotional distress, that is, that you have completed the first and second points. Trying to start by lecturing your child will not be effective. Even if what your child tells you, or the reason for their discomfort, seems insignificant to you, you need to give it the importance it has for them. After tuning in to their emotions (right hemisphere), you can then redirect their behavior with your words (left hemisphere). For example, if your little one has noticed that you have been spending more time in front of the computer than with them lately and has interpreted this as meaning that you don't love them, you could explain to them in a logical way how hard you try to be with them, and that this past month, due to that important work you had to finish, it had not been possible to spend as much time with them as you would have liked. Be sure to make a plan so that you can spend quality time together in the coming days. If the child is preverbal, that is, still very young and unable to communicate with words, you can tell them what you have perceived and also draw up a plan: "Honey, I see that you have been crying a lot lately. I think you are telling me that you want to spend more time with me. I'm going to organize everything so that we can go to the park for a little while every day." Even if your little one does not understand the meaning of your words, they will perceive the tone and emotion of what you are saying.

I want to close this chapter by reminding you that every conflict or problem is a learning opportunity. If at any point during the day you find yourself asking "What can I do to get my child to change?", change the question to "What is my child trying to tell me with their behavior and how can I help them?"

Notes

1 Berne, E. (2014). *Más allá de juegos y guiones*. Compiled by C. Steiner. Seville: Editorial Jeder.
2 Edwards, G. (2011). *El Triángulo Dramático de Karpman. Cómo trascender los roles de Perseguidor, Salvador o Víctima*. Móstoles: Gaia Ediciones.
3 Edwards, G. (2011), *El Triángulo Dramático de Karpman. Cómo trascender los roles de Perseguidor, Salvador o Víctima*. Móstoles: Gaia Ediciones.
4 Siegel, D., and Bryson, T.P. (2020). *El poder de la presencia. Cómo la presencia de los padres moldea el cerebro de los hijos y configura las personas que llegarán a ser*. Barcelona: Alba.
5 Seligman, M. (2016). *Niños optimistas*. Barcelona: Penguin Random House Grupo Editorial.

Chapter 5

Attachment and its relationship to mental health

> We have to let our children learn that there is pain in life, but that lesson must be accompanied by the deep awareness that they will never have to suffer alone.
>
> (Siegel and Bryson)

Researchers have discovered, with great interest, that adults who had parents who fostered secure attachment during their childhood, by being proactive in meeting not only their physical but also their emotional needs, are adults who are generally more likely to enjoy good relationships, regulate their emotions, develop their intellectual potential, feel respected, and have the ability to respect others.

As discussed, John Bowlby argued that mental health involves the successful management of conflicts. This same author, a pioneer of "attachment theory," was already talking, in 1940, about attachment behavior as a biological function as important as eating, and that its purpose is to direct the person toward seeking protection from someone they know who will be willing to help them unconditionally. In other words, when we are born, we are already programmed to attach ourselves to a significant other, and this is a biological survival response. That significant other cannot be just anyone, it is mostly those who really matter to us. Bowlby states the following: "Attachment behavior is any form of behavior that results in achieving or maintaining proximity to another clearly identified individual who is considered best able to cope with the world. This is most obvious when the person is frightened, tired, or ill, and feels relieved by comfort and care".[1]

> Our children are born completely dependent; it is our responsibility to provide them with the care and attention they need so that they can grow and thrive in life.

As discussed previously, from infancy, children construct an idea about themselves and the world around them based on the responses they receive from their caregivers to their physical, emotional, social, and cognitive needs. If the

DOI: 10.4324/9781003784487-5

caregiver's response is contingent, that is, if most of the time the caregiver responds sufficiently well to the child's expressed need, then the child creates an image of himself as someone capable of asking for help when needed and an idea of the other as someone close and trustworthy to whom he can turn when he needs help.

Whether the caregiver's response is consistent or not, the child creates thought patterns and coping mechanisms in order to adapt as best as possible as a means of survival. The difference between the two is that the child who has had a caregiver who is attuned and responds sufficiently well to their needs will be more likely to cope with life's vicissitudes from a platform of optimal security because they have had an attachment figure to whom they have bonded securely, providing them with sufficient emotional resources to feel capable.

In this regard, I would like to cite a well-known study conducted in 1977 in Baltimore by psychologist Mary Ainsworth to study attachment behavior and exploratory behavior in children and a balance of both when the children were at home with their mothers and when they were in a test situation in a space other than their home (laboratory). This study was conducted with a sample of 23 children aged 12 months, obtaining data from prolonged observation sessions in which the care, attention, and response of the mother to her child's needs during the first year of life were recorded. This research is often referred to as the "strange situation." It consisted of establishing two moments of separation between the child and his mother to analyze his attitude and exploratory behavior under the stressful situation of being separated from his mother. In other words, they wanted to observe how the child behaved with and without his mother both at home and in a space outside the home, the laboratory, which they called the "slightly strange test situation."

Based on the results obtained, the children were classified into four groups, taking into account three criteria:

1 Whether they explored a lot or a little when they were with their mother and when they were without her.
2 How they interacted with their mother when she was present, when she left, and, above all, when she returned.
3 How the mother responded to reassure her child when she returned to the room.

Group 1 (children with secure attachment): There was a group of 23 children who exhibited very active exploratory behavior, especially in the presence of their mother. As soon as they entered the room, they began to play with the toys that were there, and when they noticed that their mother was trying to leave surreptitiously, they began to cry and stopped playing. The crying continued as a form of protest, demanding their mother's return and focusing solely on her absence, losing all interest in the game. As soon as she returned, the child approached her seeking comfort and found a proactive and contingent response from his mother, who comforted and reassured him with her gaze, her presence, her security, and her words. Once the child calmed down, he returned to playing and exploring the room with great enthusiasm.

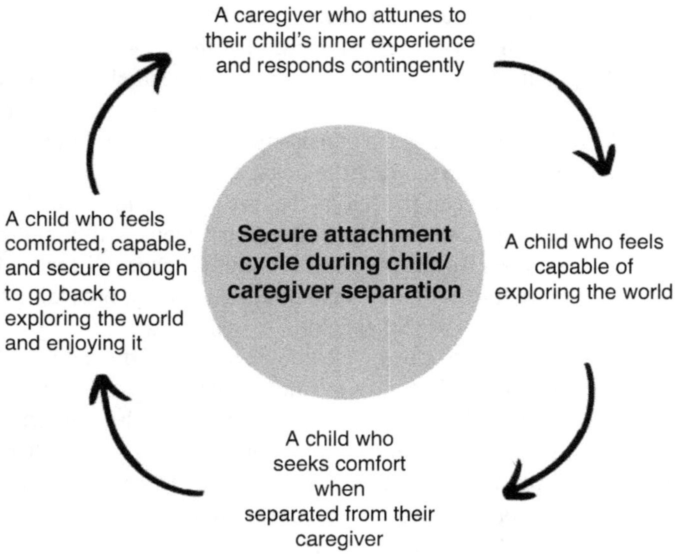

Group 2 (children with anxious-ambivalent attachment): They appeared anxious when their mother moved and cried when she left. When she returned, they had difficulty calming down and appeared both sad and angry. The mother showed neither the capacity nor the ability to hetero-regulate her child, so even though the child was now with her, he found it difficult to explore and play again.

Group 3 (children with avoidant-type insecure attachment): These children seemed indifferent when their mother left the room. When she returned, although they appeared sad, they avoided closeness and contact with her, hiding their emotions. Attachment experts say that this is a mechanism that the child uses in order to remain attached to their attachment figure. This is probably because when they feel sad and cry, they are often reprimanded and rejected by their attachment figures. For a young child, staying attached to their caregiver will always be a priority, even if this means "silencing" their emotional world.

Group 4 (children with disorganized insecure attachment): I should mention that this concept, categorized as "disorganized insecure attachment," was coined by Mary Main and her colleagues at the University of California based on this same "strange situation" study.

In the test, this group of children were passive when they entered the room and explored the available toys very little. Instead, they alternately approached and moved away from their mothers, choosing to suck their thumbs or rock themselves. Experts describe this response as chaotic and disorganized. When the mother returned, the children displayed paradoxical behavior: they approached her for comfort but then backed away and ignored her presence. Attachment experts explain that these behaviors are linked to how caregivers respond to the child.

Caregivers may react to the child's frustration by frightening them or by failing to help them regulate, thereby intensifying the child's fear and anxiety.

As we can see, attachment behavior begins as a response to a fundamentally biological need: to feel protected, connected, and cared for by our attachment figures. It eventually becomes a set of mental patterns and models through which we perceive, interpret, generate beliefs, and relate to ourselves and the world around us, and this can continue even if mom or dad are no longer present.

5.1 Why secure attachment is important for children

Hartzell and Siegel (2019) say that attachment is an innate brain system designed to keep kids safe, leading them to (1) seek closeness with their parents, (2) turn to them in times of distress as a source of comfort and safe haven, and (3) internalize the relationship with their parents as a secure base internal model.[2]

When a baby is born, they are completely dependent on their caregivers; they cannot take care of themselves in order to survive. Having an adult who feeds them, provides care, attends to their needs, and is able to perceive, interpret, and respond to their physical and emotional needs is key to the child's sense of security and ability to thrive. When the child's natural environment is filled with that care and their inner sense of well-being is maintained consistently because their primary caregiver is close, loving, and affectionate when they demand care and attention, the child learns that this response from their caregiver is predictable and reliable. This gives them security, allowing them to create an internal schema of themselves as someone capable of asking for help and of their caregiver as a secure base from which they can explore the world and to which they can return when they need to. Rafa Guerrero puts it this way: "The two basic pillars of secure attachment are, on the one hand, bonding and, on the other hand, autonomy. There are other aspects that are synonymous or similar to bonding, such as affection, protection, intimacy, security, etc. Anything that protects the child will serve as a synonym".[3]

Research on attachment shows the significant influence of the parent-child relationship on children's relationships with their peers. Depending on the type of attachment we form with them, we provide them with greater or lesser security as they explore the world, greater or lesser ability to manage frustration and stress, their skills for regulating emotions, the narrative or internal discourse they construct about themselves, and, therefore, the quality of the relationships they establish at each stage of their lives. Therefore, talking about the importance of fostering secure attachment means, at the same time, caring for and protecting the mental health of our children.

Before continuing to talk about the importance of attachment for our children's mental health, I want to pause here and say something that I think is very important to encourage you as a caregiver. When we read about the great influence that the way we relate to our children has, we can feel both satisfied and concerned. We may feel satisfied because we recognize some things we have done well, but we may also feel concerned.

We may think something like, "Well, I haven't done so badly. I think I'm on the right track and taking care of my child's mental health," or we may feel worried as we reflect on our parenting and notice a knot in our stomach and throat when we realize that we have made many mistakes along the way and that these may be affecting our child's mental health. I want you to know that I see you, I understand you, and I embrace you. This book is not meant to make you feel guilty, but to encourage you to take responsibility and help your children with the most valuable resources you have, because you do have them. You just need to learn to see them and redirect them. I want to end this brief note with a fact mentioned by Hartzell and Siegel (2019): "Research shows that relationships with parents can change over time, just as children's attachments change. That means it's never too late to make positive changes in the lives of young children".[4]

Most of us do not consider that every experience our children have, based on what they receive from the outside world, generates reactions within them. This is what we know as "internal experience." What children experience internally provokes a response that is expressed through bodily sensations, emotions, thoughts or cognitions, and actions. These are the four responses common to all experiences.

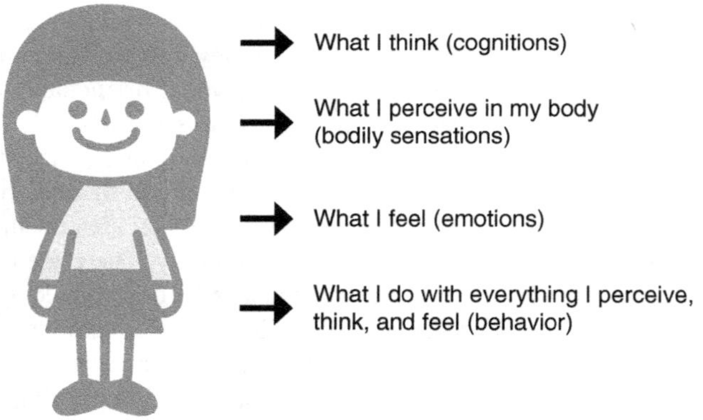

The key to helping children progress while fostering secure attachment lies in tuning into their inner world, accurately interpreting their reactions, and providing them with appropriate support as they navigate the emotions that the experience may have triggered. We refer to the latter as "heteroregulation." When we tune into their inner world, interpret their reactions appropriately, and provide appropriate emotional support (heteroregulation), we are being contingent in our response, and we can then speak of an optimal life experience. Let's look at an example of how this might sound.

Let's imagine that you have planned your child's birthday party. As part of the preparations, you have hired a clown with the best of intentions to liven up the party and entertain the little ones. The moment the clown enters the room, he walks over to where you are standing with your child in his typical costume, approaches him, and says in that characteristic voice, "Whose birthday is it today?" Your child clings to you with all his might, looks at you for refuge because of the fear he is feeling throughout his body, and from there begins to cry inconsolably.

Your child may not have had an experience like this with a clown, but they may have been frightened by loud fireworks, a dog barking or coming too close to them, witnessing a fight, or any other experience that had a strong emotional impact on them. Keep in mind that the event itself is not as important as how your child perceives and experiences it.

The mother who has planned this birthday party, and who intends to foster a secure attachment with her son in her daily life, decides to carry out three fundamental tasks in order to connect with her son's inner experience by providing him with the support he needs at that moment: (1) she shows closeness by connecting emotionally with her son and conveying comfort. We convey comfort primarily through our attitude rather than our words. A powerful tool for this is to establish physical contact with our child: touching their shoulder, offering a hug, holding their hands, and rubbing their back are ways in which we are non-verbally conveying that we are there with them. In addition, studies show that receiving or providing physical contact with someone significant to us decreases cortisol (stress hormone) levels and increases the production of pleasure hormones such as oxytocin, and good mood hormones such as dopamine and serotonin. In addition to this, maintain an affectionate gaze that conveys security. If, at that moment, the mother is holding the child in her arms but looking at them disapprovingly, the child's nervous system will remain dysregulated because the mother's disapproving gaze becomes as threatening as the clown in front of them. The explanation for this is that the child's sensory system perceives the mother's facial expressions and registers them as threatening, which activates their defensive and reactive circuits, further intensifying the child's fear and the mother's frustration and anger. So remember:

It is essential to train our gaze: The compassion you convey to your child with a gaze is literally a caress to their nervous system. They still need exactly the same support they received from you when they were a newborn and did not have the words to tell you they needed you, and yet you understood by cradling and comforting them.

1 Legitimize their emotions by empathizing with their discomfort. Legitimizing means accepting emotions as they arise without labeling them as good or bad. We legitimize when we refuse to minimize the experience that our child or anyone else has had. If this mother had not legitimized her son, she would have said something like, "Son, it's not that big of a deal, it's just a clown," "You told me you wanted a clown party, and now you're crying like a baby," or she might have even kindly invalidated his emotions by saying something like, "Don't cry, sweetie. Let's go get some ice cream so you'll stop crying."

   Without realizing it, parents repeatedly invalidate their children's emotional experiences, sending them the message that what they are going through and feeling is exaggerated and irrelevant. So, to validate her son's feelings, this mother said to him, "You're scared, aren't you? You didn't expect the clown to appear suddenly." When you do this, accompanied by the first point, you are conveying the message to your child that you understand them and that you deeply understand why they feel that way. We call this "empathy." And we can convey empathy when we understand that, even though what has happened may seem small, insignificant, or silly to us, it is very meaningful to our child and deserves our understanding. So, once you have done all this, you can continue to translate the experience, as described in point 3.

2 Verbally translate what happened. When you do this, you are helping your child connect their right hemisphere (emotional) with their left hemisphere (words), and we know this process as "integration." Since the child in the story is young, his mother took it upon herself to describe what had happened, doing so as if it were a picture in front of her, with her being responsible for conveying what she saw. So she said to him, "You're scared of the clown. You were playing with your friends and suddenly the clown appeared, coming very quickly toward you and talking very loudly. That's why you ran straight to me and I took you in my arms to help you feel safe, and then you started to calm down little by little." When we put the experience that has impacted the child into order, we help them make sense of what they have experienced by integrating their emotions, thoughts, and actions with their body. This mother emphasized the latter, that she helped him feel better, ensuring that the feeling of safety was part of the child's experience and narrative.

The cycle of heteroregulation

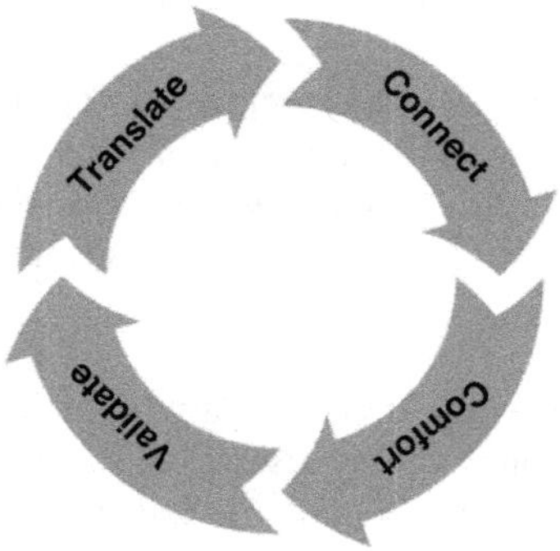

Repeating experiences like the one above, in which we accompany our children with compassion, empathy, and closeness and show them that difficult situations can bend them but not break them, have a profound impact on their lives and on how they relate to themselves and others.

5.2 Adult attachment. My own style of attachment

If everything we experienced in our childhood remained anecdotal, many popular beliefs such as "they hit me and I wasn't traumatized" would make sense. The truth is that it doesn't work that way. The attachment style built with our primary caregivers shapes how we see ourselves and the world and, of course, how we perceive and relate to others.

As children, we learned from our interactions with our parents whether our needs would be met, and this then shaped how we feel about ourselves and others. We were very vulnerable at birth and completely dependent on what our caregivers did for us. Whenever we had a physiological or emotional need, they usually responded in a specific way that also conveyed a mental model of what it means to relate to others.

For example, when we were afraid and cried at night because we didn't want to sleep alone, we had an emotional need for protection and comfort. The usual way our caregivers responded to this need instilled in us a specific belief:

> "When I'm scared, I know I can call Mom to calm down," or the opposite: "When I'm scared, I can't cry because they scold me and I feel even more scared."

Each of these experiences was lived through the four elements common to all experiences:

- Physical sensations: dilated pupils, sweating, and rapid heartbeat.
- Emotions: fear.
- Thought: "I am able to ask for help when I need it and I have someone to turn to" versus "I cannot ask for help, I have no one to turn to."
- Actions: "I cry to find comfort" versus "I suppress my crying because no one will come to me or to avoid being scolded."

Although we may not consciously remember many of these experiences because we were very young, our bodies stored part of those moments in the form of bodily sensations, emotions, and perceptions (implicit memories). That is why we sometimes react to certain situations without finding a logical explanation for why we scream, hit, or insult others. That event could be a "trigger" for that unconscious emotional memory.

It is normal for you to respond the way you do; it is part of your life story. If your caregivers adequately met your needs, not only physical but also emotional, social, and cognitive, you are likely to have developed a more adaptive belief system regarding your relationships with others and yourself, and your narrative about your experiences is likely to be coherent, complete, integrated, and effective.

The emotional bonds we create with our attachment figures while interacting with them ("I am capable, I can ask for help" versus "the world is a hostile place, I cannot trust others enough") have become our "internal compass," also called our "representational system," through which we relate to our partner, coworkers, friends, and, of course, our children. We unconsciously reproduce the same pattern of behavior because it is what feels familiar and safe to us based on the signals sent by our nervous system. Remember this: your glasses are neither good nor bad. Your response is biologically correct.

So, the way we tell our own story and the emphasis we place on different details of those experiences may convey the view we have of ourselves and the world around us.

Next, I will provide information that may help us see our adult attachment style. However, I want to mention that it is very important not to try to rigidly pigeonhole yourself into one of these four categories, as if it were a personality test or something similar. It is normal to find aspects of different attachment styles within yourself. This is because, as children, the different attachment patterns we developed depended on the quality of our relationships with the different adults we interacted with. You may have had a secure attachment with your mother and an insecure avoidant attachment with your father, or vice versa.

That said, the idea is that this information, rather than pigeonholing you into one type of attachment or another, is intended to help you gain a greater understanding of yourself and your life experiences and to work more consciously and intentionally on yourself and your relationship with your children, fostering secure attachment.

Secure attachment: Having a secure attachment style could be related to the fact that you had caregivers who understood and adequately met both your physiological and emotional needs. In other words, they were contingent in the way they met your needs. You were cold, so they wrapped you up warm; you were afraid, so they stayed with you; you felt angry, so they helped you feel better with their presence. They were not perfect parents, but, as Winnicott says, they were sufficiently good parents.

Growing up in an environment where you mostly perceived and received attention, security, and understanding while interacting with your caregivers may have built within you an internal sense that your caregiver was your source of security and trust, someone you could turn to without fear, even when you made mistakes. You learned to feel valued, accepted, and loved for who you were and not exclusively for what you did or did not do. A person with a secure attachment style tends to be confident in themselves and their abilities. They feel capable of saying no and setting boundaries in their relationships.

Avoidant attachment: Having an avoidant attachment style may reflect a childhood marked by emotional neglect and an internal feeling of being constantly rejected or humiliated by your caregivers. These children assumed that their emotional needs would not be met by their primary caregivers, so they learned to "meet" them themselves in some way. Parents with avoidant attachment are very insensitive to the emotional signals their children send them. Therefore, children try to adapt to the situation by avoiding emotional connection and closeness to their parents as a survival mechanism. Adults with this avoidant attachment style often feel uncomfortable with closeness, but deep down, they long for it. Closeness may feel dangerous, unsafe, or uncomfortable for them, as they have learned that independence is the "place" that gives them the most security. As a result, they may avoid making new friends, or they may not like others very much and become attached to themselves. This can be quite lonely in the long run, leading them to feel disconnected from others and their own inner world. They "shut down" their feelings as a defense mechanism to protect themselves. This happens on an unconscious level. In parenting, parents with this attachment style tend to have an authoritarian parenting style.

Anxious-ambivalent attachment: This type of attachment is very common, especially if, as a child, you felt that communication with your parents was inconsistent and sometimes intrusive, leaving you with a persistent feeling of not knowing what to expect from them. Sometimes you felt that they were making an effort to connect with you, and then, soon afterward, they would swing to the other extreme of indifference. This ambivalence often creates a feeling of insecurity in the relationship between the child and their caregiver. An adult with anxious-ambivalent attachment may be afraid to say no for fear of disappointing others; they may find it difficult to set boundaries in their relationships and do their best to earn the trust and admiration of others. They often find it difficult to be alone, emotionally and physically. They tend to neglect their own needs and desires in order to please others. Parents with an anxious-ambivalent attachment style are often known as "overprotective" parents.

Disorganized attachment: This attachment style is like a "mix" of avoidant and ambivalent attachment. People with this attachment style tend to swing between anxiety and avoidance. They have a desire to get close to people, but at the same time, they may be afraid to trust them due to fear of being abandoned. It is like an internal battle between "I love you, please don't leave me" and "I hate you, get out of my life." This feeling usually stems from emotional abuse or early relational trauma, as well as past abusive relationships. Parents with this type of attachment often physically and emotionally abuse their children, often becoming both a source of protection and fear at the same time. In other words, the child grows up with the internal feeling that the person they should turn to for protection when they are afraid is the same person who causes them fear and terror: two contradictory neural pathways that are activated at the same time, which Mary Main calls "biological paradox or fear without solution."

5.2.1 Reflections on attachment

You may be wondering whether your attachment style condemns you to repeat the same parenting patterns with your children, or if the consequences of insecure attachment will condition your life and relationships forever. The answer to this is no, and scientific evidence supports this. Even people who have had childhoods marked by neglect or abuse have been able to overcome the wounds these experiences caused them when they have had the opportunity to have people close to them who provided support, encouragement, and emotional security. As Boris Cyrulnik says, an unhappy childhood does not determine your life. When you make sense of your life experiences, understanding that your behavior up to that point was your way of safeguarding yourself because that is what you learned in childhood as a way to protect yourself and survive, then little by little you can learn to be more compassionate and kind to yourself. You can learn to "renarrate" your life, changing your internal dialogue to one that is more complete, integrated, effective, and coherent. Instead of sounding like "I'm just very anxious," this new narrative might be constructed as follows: "I grew up surrounded by people who were overwhelmed with their own problems and insensitive to my needs. Growing up in that environment, I felt that I had to solve things on my own and that it was best not to ask for help. That inner feeling led me to experience high levels of stress, which remain with me to this day."

And what is the difference between one narrative and another?

In the first narrative, you have constructed a belief about yourself based on an adaptive, survival response that was necessary at that point in your life but is not based on who you really are. In the second, you have constructed an integrated, complete, coherent, and effective narrative that allows you to understand that what you have experienced has led you to feel and act anxiously until today.

What you had to do to adapt to that moment in your life is not a trait of your personality; I repeat: it is a response that was adaptive at the time because you were in a very sensitive period and needed to feel connected in order to survive. During those years, feeling that you belonged was more important than looking after your emotional well-being.

Thinking that you were born an anxious, controlling, fearful, or compliant person is very understandable, because when you have experienced high levels of stress since childhood—because you felt lonely or misunderstood, because you were perhaps afraid of being punished or beaten, because of the constant fights and arguments at home, or because one of your caregivers died—it is as if an internal turmoil has been "turned on" ever since and has been with you all these years, leading you to the conclusion that you were born that way.

Feeling constantly "held hostage" by your emotions is a sign that you have been carrying a heavy burden of fear, guilt, anger, and shame for many years without really being able to process it; it does not mean that you have a "flaw" from birth or a defining personality trait.

So, if you are one of those people who has thought, "I am very anxious," or "parenting has made me a more anxious person," then you can begin by working through the stress you've been carrying for years. This means giving voice to what you've silenced, whether because the context required you to be silent or because you disassociated from those experiences and left them out of your consciousness. This can be a starting point for building an integrated, complete, coherent, and effective narrative.

Embracing everything we are can be a very arduous and difficult task at first, but ultimately it allows us to accept ourselves compassionately and improves our interpersonal connections. The coherence of one's life story is only possible when issues from the past are integrated with our present history, while looking toward the future.[5]

Our attachment style is not something to be ashamed of. It was a useful way to survive during a very sensitive period of our lives—childhood. Realizing this can help us understand why we see the world the way we do and why we relate to others the way we do; how the way we related to our caregivers not only conditioned us at that time, but has also shaped our lives, perhaps even to this day. From there, we can take small steps and make changes that will lead to significant growth in every area of our lives.

5.3 Does attachment parenting mean secure attachment?

If we go on social media, we can read a lot of information urging us to "parent with attachment." And this is a concept that, in my opinion, we need to clarify.

It is impossible to parent without attachment. We have already seen that attachment behavior is a response to a biological human need that drives us to bond with a significant other, especially mom and dad, in order to protect ourselves and survive. So, using the expression "attachment parenting" as a synonym for "secure attachment parenting" is not accurate.

Secure attachment can only be established when the caregiver-child relationship, or the relationship with another primary caregiver, maintains communication based on five fundamental parameters: consistency, reliability, responsiveness, clear boundaries, and a non-intrusive approach, all under the umbrella of assertive parenting, whose starting point is unconditional acceptance.[6] This type of contingent interaction between the child and their caregivers provides children with a continuous sense of experiences in which they feel safe, connected, understood, and protected, which has a positive impact on their emotional well-being. This emotional well-being is ultimately reflected in their ability to recognize, express, and regulate their own emotions, because there was first an adult attuned to their emotional world who helped them translate, legitimize, label, and regulate all of that emotional experience.

5.4 The five keys to becoming a secure base

A caregiver who is seen and accepted by the child as a secure base is someone whom the child perceives as a source from which to explore the world around them and to whom they can return when they need shelter, support, rest, help, comfort, connection, and security to recharge. For a child to view their attachment figure as that source or secure base, that adult must first have shown themselves to be consistent, reliable, responsive, close, and able to set clear boundaries. This task may sound impossible in practice, but remember that your job is not to be a perfect parent, but to meet your children's needs.

To understand a little more about how we can become that safe haven for our children, let's explain each of these basic parameters:

- Consistency: A consistent adult is someone who practices what they preach. When I talk about consistency in parenting, I always refer to what Teresa of Calcutta said: "Don't worry if your children don't listen to you; they watch you all day long." And I conclude that thought by saying: "Don't set a limit for your child that you are not capable of assuming yourself first. Because, in order to teach, we need to model." How inconsistent is a parent who hits their child, pretending that this will teach the child not to hit others. How inconsistent it is when we yell at our children to stop yelling. Families, in order to teach our children something, we must first have mastered it ourselves. If we want our children to speak respectfully to others, they must first feel respected themselves. If we want our children to be able to deal effectively with their own frustration, they need to see us first dealing effectively with our own frustration. Our emotional state influences the emotional state of our children, and our mirror neuron system is responsible for this. Let me explain briefly. Have you ever been watching a movie and suddenly found yourself crying when you saw that mother in tears because she had just given birth to her baby and was holding him to her chest? Or have you ever suddenly seen someone yawn and found yourself yawning too? Well, mirror neurons, located in Broca's area—which is related to language—and in the posterior parietal cortex, are responsible for this. These neurons are activated mainly in three situations: when an action is performed, when we see someone else performing an action, and when we mentally represent ourselves performing an action.

  An example of the latter is when you read about yawning a few seconds ago, and even though you haven't seen anyone yawn at this precise moment, you probably feel the urge to do so just by imagining it. Daniel Goleman compares mirror neurons to "neural Wi-Fi." Van der Kolk says that we not only pick up on another person's movements, but also their emotional state and intentions. When people are in sync, they tend to adopt the same posture or sit in the same way, and their voices end up adopting the same rhythm.

  That's why consistency is essential for secure attachment, and for life itself, because your child will learn that they are important to you and that they can turn to you, not because they are your child, but because of the way you treat them.

  Is what you say consistent with what you do? When you tell your child, "Trust me, even if you make a mistake," is that really true? Can they approach you without fear? If so, the foundation on which you are building your relationship with your child is consistent. If not, you can start putting it into practice today. Sometimes we just need to hear again how important it is to practice what we preach.

- Reliability: A reliable caregiver is precisely someone you can turn to in the midst of a storm, knowing that they will support you and not reject you; a caregiver who, even without having all the answers or solutions, is committed to your well-being and protection. They are someone who is not against you, but on your side.
- Responsive or contingent: A contingent caregiver is one who adequately meets the child's needs, although that does not mean giving the child what they want; in the last chapter, we will talk about the 17 emotional needs and the difference between a need and a desire. When a caregiver is responsive, the child grows up with the feeling that they are not alone in the world and with the internalized idea that they are someone capable of asking for help when they need it, because they have someone capable of providing it at that moment.
- Non-intrusive closeness: A close caregiver is one who is close without being controlling; one who accompanies the child when the storm rages, but at the same time allows spaces where the child is able to see their own resources. A caregiver who provides roots, says "count on me," and at the same time gives wings helps the child develop the necessary resources to deal with the situation on their own. This is a caregiver who "pushes" when they see that the child has the necessary skills to resolve certain situations on their own, but who "cushions" when they realize that their child is not ready to deal with certain situations. Your 6-year-old may not yet feel ready to strike up a conversation on her own when she goes to a birthday party, and she will need your company to say "hello." And your 8-year-old may already feel ready to sleep away from home at summer camp and just needs you to give her that "push" by saying, "I know you can spend these three nights sleeping with your friends at camp." Taking that leap of faith can give her that inner feeling of "I did it," and that's a wonderful ingredient for building healthy self-esteem. Whatever it is, a close, consistent, and reliable caregiver will not ask the child to figure something out on their own when they are not yet ready to do so.
- Clear boundaries: A caregiver who sets clear boundaries knows that their child needs to know what is and is not expected of them. They are not afraid to say no, because their goal is not to make their child happy at all costs.

Above all else, be careful. This does not mean leaving them alone to deal with their frustration, anger, or any emotional distress, hoping that they will "become stronger." That is called "emotional neglect." Instead, what matters is allowing them to weather the storm with us by their side, teaching them, through our unconditional love and presence, to tolerate frustration when things don't turn out as they expect.

Let me emphasize this point. It is not true that saying no to your children will traumatize them; it is not true that, solely because of the no, they will grow up with a limited and narrow mindset. As with many aspects of positive parenting, there has been a lot of confusion about the use of no. A message can be distorted by word of mouth and end up losing its original meaning.

It is true that you can use "no" to set limits for your child, especially when it comes to their safety, health, and respect for others. It is true that you can use "no" without overusing it. Don't wear it out! It is true that you should use it while also expressing what you expect to happen. It is true that children, and adults too, understand better when we give instructions in a positive way. The classic example is, if I say "don't think about a white elephant," you are probably thinking about a white elephant right now. That's true!

I am in favor of using "no," but only while taking into account everything I mentioned earlier. And why am I in favor of using "no"? Because setting limits using "no" teaches our children to be adults who respect when "no means no" in the face of any kind of abuse; because we have demonized it so much, to the point of creating the confusion that assertive parenting is parenting without limits; and because life itself will put many "no's" in our path, and I am convinced that our home is the best place to train our children to tolerate the frustration that this generates.

Five points to keep in mind:

1 Be consistent: As I said before, don't set a limit that you're not willing to enforce yourself.
2 Be a role model: Your children will learn more from what they see you do than from what you tell them to do.
3 Be clear: If you know in advance that you are going to say no, then avoid saying things like, "Well, I don't know; I'll think about it."
4 Be fair: If you promised something and suddenly something happened that made you angry, don't blame your child for your reaction. Take responsibility for managing your anger.
5 Kindly accompany the emotions that this limit generates in your child.

We have discussed the five parameters for a secure base, and I would also like to conclude this section with something I learned from my teacher Begoña Aznárez, also discussed in Chapter 4. The foundation on which these five parameters are based is the unconditional gaze. It is through the gaze of the caregiver that the child constructs themselves, narrates themselves, and learns to look at themselves and others. From that same gaze, the child, later as an adult, perceives the world, interprets it, generates beliefs, and acts based on them. If the child has had a consistent, reliable, responsive, and close caregiver who knew how to set clear boundaries, it is very likely that they have received a gaze that will help them create complete beliefs and narratives about who they are. But if their caregiver was negligent in this task, it is likely that the belief generated will be that of someone incapable, defective, and unwanted, with an incomplete, incoherent, ineffective, and disintegrated narrative that sometimes reads as "I am who I am because of the blows I received," when in reality it could be: "I am who I am despite the undeserved blows I received in my childhood."

Notes

1 Bowlby, J. (1989). *Una base segura: aplicaciones clínicas de la teoría del apego*. Barcelona: Paidós Ibérica.
2 Hartzell, M., and Siegel, D. (2019). *Ser padres conscientes*. Barcelona: Ediciones La Llave.
3 Guerrero, R. (2020b). *Educar en el vínculo*. Barcelona: Plataforma Actual.
4 Hartzell, M., and Siegel, D. (2019). *Ser padres conscientes*. Barcelona: Ediciones La Llave.
5 Hartzell, M., and Siegel, D. (2019). *Ser padres conscientes*. Barcelona: Ediciones La Llave.
6 I learned these five parameters for secure attachment during my training in brief psychotherapy with children and adolescents under the guidance of Begoña Aznárez, president of the Spanish Society of Psychosomatic Medicine and Psychotherapy.

Chapter 6

Understanding psychological trauma

> It is traumatic for any human being to have to remain silent about anything that happens to them and that has an emotional impact on them.
>
> (Begoña Aznárez)

People often ask me, "Milena, what is trauma?" And I find much of the answer in the way it is expressed by Begoña Aznárez, whose quote opens this chapter, and from whom I have learned firsthand much of what I know about trauma, attachment, and family systems.

If we look at the definition of "trauma" as specified by the Royal Spanish Academy, we find first of all that "trauma" derives from the Greek word, which means "wound," and it includes three definitions:

1 *Emotional shock that causes lasting damage to the unconscious.*
2 *Strong and lasting negative emotion or impression.*
3 *Med. Lasting injury caused by a mechanical agent, usually external.*

In these three definitions provided by the Royal Spanish Academy, we see that there is one word common to all of them, and that is "lasting."

As we will see throughout this chapter, psychological trauma is not determined only by the emotional impact of an event. It is also shaped by how long the experience lasts, how repeatedly and alone the person endures it, and whether they have the internal and external resources needed to cope.

Trauma theory usually divided into two categories: simple trauma and complex trauma. This distinction is made not because one type of trauma is greater than the other, but in order to better understand the origin of the suffering of those who experienced it and, among other things, to know the different intervention protocols to be used therapeutically.

Simple trauma is usually associated with a single event whose emotional impact is readily recognized, such as a tsunami, earthquake, car accident, the death of a loved one, kidnapping, sexual abuse, or rape. When a person remains emotionally

DOI: 10.4324/9781003784487-6

affected by such an event to the point that they cannot function adaptively in daily life, this is often described as simple trauma. It is generally linked to a recent traumatic episode whose significant psychological impact is clear.

However, studies, psychological consultations, and fieldwork continue to show every day that what is traumatic for a person is not only the event itself, but also the loneliness with which that person has experienced that event. It is the absence of someone close to them who legitimizes their experience, provides emotional support, and serves as a reliable place where that person feels safe and secure enough to talk and think about what happened.

Therefore, when we talk about complex trauma, it is extremely important to bear in mind that it occurs at a time of extreme vulnerability, such as childhood. For a long period of time, the child has felt completely invisible, silenced, and alone, experiencing situations that tend to be minimized socially and situations in which their suffering is denied, ignored, and invalidated. This suffering, if it is not translated, seen, and addressed, is perpetuated into adulthood as a result of childhood emotional abandonment, situations that caused them great fear and that they could not share with anyone, and life experiences in which they may have felt humiliated or ashamed.

I usually explain these two concepts as I learned them from Begoña.

We talk about simple trauma when we refer to a situation that we did not expect but that suddenly appears and hits us with such intensity that it has the power to break us such as the death of a loved one, witnessing a robbery, having to be confined to our homes from one day to the next, undergoing an emergency operation due to serious illness, or experiencing the explosion of a volcano in our area of residence, and so on. And we talk about complex trauma when the experience we go through is not usually as shocking at first, but when lived every day, over a sustained period of time, and without a responsive adult capable of sustaining all that impact, it also ends up breaking us inside as if we had received an unexpected blow.

This is because complex trauma generally develops during childhood, as we mentioned earlier, when human beings are the most vulnerable. When your father or mother defended and used physical punishment as a means of correction, when emotional neglect, power abuse, and a constant feeling of vulnerability were your daily bread. All of this undoubtedly left its mark on you.

I want you to imagine that this is your head and that you receive a powerful impact. The blow is so strong that it immediately breaks your head.

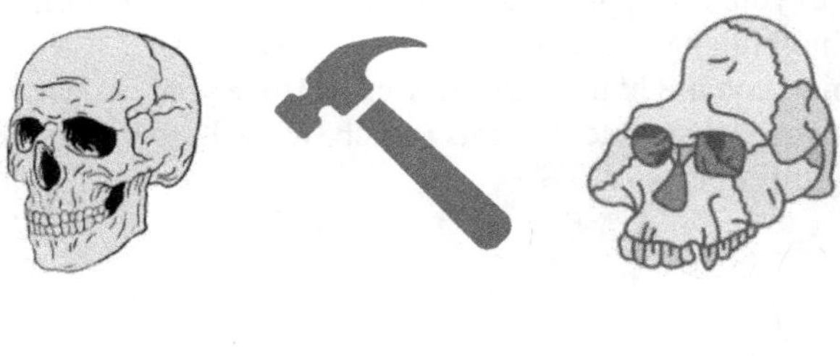

Now I want you to imagine again that this is your head, but instead of receiving a strong impact, it receives a drop every day, slowly, every second, every moment. That drop apparently does no harm. But what would happen if it continued to fall like this for many years without respite?

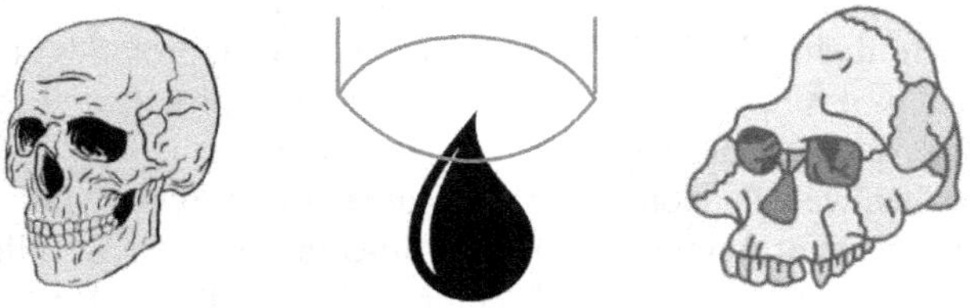

In the first case, it seems obvious that such a strong blow would break your head, right? Well, we can liken that blow to what we know as "simple trauma"; as we have already said, no single dispute can affect a person emotionally. It is such a shocking experience that it has the capacity to break you on the spot and attract the attention of those around you.

In the second case, it is a drop of water that seems harmless but is so persistent over the years that it ends up breaking your head anyway. We can liken that drop to what we know as "complex trauma." Something that many do not believe can affect a child's soul. For example, that constant feeling of abandonment, that daily abuse of power justified by the idea "spare the rod and spoil the child," that "timely blow" that is so often defended, or those hurtful words that lacerate the soul:

"I'm going to give you a good reason to cry."

That hole that forms causes terrible pain. It creates terrible feeling of emptiness. It acts like a black hole that swallows everything and gives no respite. It is the daily protagonist of small but significant internal dramas and, on many occasions, external ones as well. It is a torment that has always been present and is a constant companion. People try to silence it by filling it in different ways: with food, drink, substances that are more or less toxic, people who are also toxic to a greater or lesser extent, work, collectibles, etc."[1]

I close this chapter by emphasizing the idea that psychological trauma is not only about what happened to us but also about what did not happen. It is also about that lack of empathy, listening, and the possibility of talking, crying, and venting in a safe place. What needs of yours or your child's have gone unseen or unmet? What experiences of yours or your child's have had to be silenced, turned away from, and treated as if nothing had happened?

At this point, you might think that any experience your child has or that you have had could become traumatic. For this reason, we will devote the following section to answering this question.

6.1 The physiological response in optimal and traumatic conditions

We are all born with an information processing system that helps us process all those experiences that have had an emotional impact on us. This system serves to integrate what has happened so that we can adapt to our daily lives again and function normally.

I want to start by explaining how our brain responds optimally to a dangerous situation, and to do so, I will draw on the explanation provided by Bessel van der Kolk in his book *The Body Keeps the Score* (published in Spanish as *El cuerpo lleva la cuenta*).

Let's start by using this doll to illustrate how humans process information.

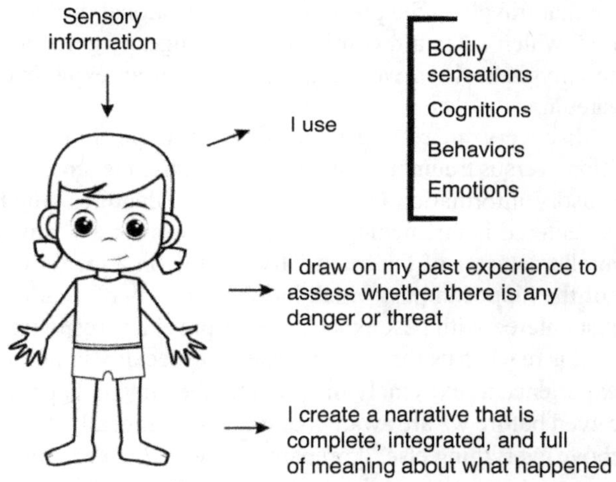

All sensory information from our external world enters us through our eyes, nose, ears, and skin. At this point, it is worth recalling the five senses we learned about in school (taste, touch, sight, hearing, and smell). When information from the world around us enters through our senses, the first place it arrives is the thalamus, a part of our brain located in our limbic zone (emotional brain) which Gerald Edelman, Nobel Prize winner in Medicine, called the "cook of the brain." The thalamus mixes all the information from our perceptions to prepare a very homogeneous autobiographical soup, an integrated and coherent experience; "this is what is happening to me."[2] Subsequently, the sensations produced travel along two pathways, one longer and one shorter: the shorter pathway leads to the amygdala (the part of the brain that informs us whether what we perceive from the outside poses a threat to our survival), and toward the frontal lobes, the longer pathway, that is, the area of the brain behind our forehead that allows us to be fully aware of what is happening. It is our prefrontal cortex that allows us to regulate ourselves and adapt so that we can function optimally in our daily lives.

Imagine you are lying in bed, and suddenly you touch a large spider-shaped object with your hand. This information has entered you through your sense of touch, and then reached the thalamus and subsequently your cerebral amygdala. From there, it went to the corresponding cortex, which, in this case, was the somatosensory cortex, which informed you about the shape, size, and texture of the object you touched. You also realized that it was not a real spider, but a plastic spider because someone wanted to play a joke on you.

Neuroscientist Joseph LeDoux is known for his interesting studies on the amygdala. In fact, he was the one who discovered that once information reaches the thalamus, it travels in two directions, and not just to the prefrontal cortex as previously believed. And that other pathway he discovered is the amygdala. He also called this pathway the "downstream path," which is very fast, while he called the information that travels to the prefrontal cortex (rational or thinking brain) the "upstream path," which takes a few milliseconds longer to get there compared to the path to the amygdala when we are in the midst of an experience that is perceived as threatening.

Why is this discovery interesting in relation to the physiological response in optimal conditions versus traumatic conditions? Because the amygdala, in addition to receiving sensory information from the thalamus, identifies whether the information that has entered is threatening or not; there is a reason why Van der Kolk calls it the "smoke detector of the brain." It does this in a matter of milliseconds with the help of the hippocampus, which has the function of relating the information that has just entered with past experiences to provide a response.

When a stimulus reaches us through our senses, especially in moments when we perceive the experience as extremely threatening, the amygdala prepares our body to fight or flee even before we are aware that there is a danger. Its function is to seek our survival above everything else. It prepares us by setting us in motion so that we can take action even before we realize what is happening. Like when you realized there was a spider on your bed. On the one hand, your amygdala warned you of a possible danger and set you in motion even before your prefrontal lobes warned you that it was a toy spider and not a real one.

Since the thalamus sends sensory information in two directions, we can see how the amygdala reacts impulsively, putting us on alert, in survival mode, while our prefrontal lobes, or thinking brain, respond proactively, making us aware of what is actually happening. This teamwork is essential for our survival and adaptation, allowing us to observe what is happening, what will happen if we do x or y, and equipping us to make a conscious decision. When all this occurs, we refer to it as a physiological response under optimal conditions.

Now, although the amygdala is usually very good at detecting danger and helping us survive, being exposed repeatedly over time to situations with a high emotional impact can cause a blockage and a disconnection between the amygdala and the thalamus, which means that our amygdala becomes overexcited and takes control without our thinking brain being able to make any conscious decisions about it.

When this system (thinking brain: amygdala) does not work in harmony, we react instead of responding, automatically putting ourselves into fight-or-flight mode the moment we detect danger, even if it does not threaten our survival; for example, the incessant crying of a newborn, the disapproving look from our mother-in-law, or the constant complaining of our teenager. As Van der Kolk says, we can only get along with others when we can accurately assess whether their intentions are good or dangerous. Faulty alarm systems cause outbursts or freezes in response to harmless comments or facial expressions.[3]

The danger signals detected by the amygdala trigger the release of powerful stress hormones, such as adrenaline and cortisol, which in turn increase our heart rate, breathing, and blood pressure. All this hormone release serves to prepare us for fight or flight, and once the danger has passed, our body quickly returns to its normal state. However, when cortisol levels are high, the emotional impact exceeds our internal and external resources, and we find ourselves in a sensitive period of our lives, such as childhood, then the possibility of our body returning to its normal state is blocked, making us feel agitated, excited, anxious, and stressed.

6.2 Physical punishment, brain, and trauma

Something I am often asked in the training courses I give is what I think about punishment.

As we have already seen, boundaries are essential for building secure attachment in our relationship with our children. However, setting boundaries has nothing to do with punishing or making a child feel bad when they have made a mistake or when we want to teach them a skill they need to learn.

Every family, caregiver, and child is different, and our own history, combined with the act of raising children, can trigger so many unresolved issues from our own childhood that it can lead some parents to resort to physical punishment as a means of discipline. Honestly, I don't like to combine the word "punishment" with the word "discipline," because there is a huge gap between the two.

We have grown up with the idea that discipline means making someone else feel bad so that they learn from it. In other words, "if it doesn't hurt, they won't learn." Discipline is associated with *a heavy hand, shouting, crying, pain, stress, and fatigue.* We are not accustomed to thinking of love, affection, and closeness as resources for teaching without causing pain or fear. And the truth is that it is neither necessary nor humane to resort to physical and emotional suffering to teach children to do things differently. We can discipline by encouraging our children and being respectful and loving toward them. You can discipline and, at the same time, build a secure attachment relationship with your child.

"The word *discipline* comes directly from *the* Latin *disciplina*, which was used in the 11th century to refer to teaching, learning, and giving instructions. Thus, since its inception, *discipline* has been related to teaching."[4]

Disciplining with love does not mean letting children do whatever they want; as we have already mentioned, that is counterproductive and harmful. Disciplining with affection and assertiveness means teaching children the skills they need to learn in order to do things differently. And for that, they need you to be connected, understanding, and compassionate. Yes, discipline begins with us, and through it, we benefit our children. It starts with you and me when we feel the deep desire to yell and, instead, decide to model the emotional state we want them to mirror in that moment. It starts with you and me when we review our own history and cry what we couldn't cry and validate what no one was able to legitimize.

> Discipline begins with us when we work on our own life script and understand that our parents also made mistakes, that we don't need to continue justifying their actions and can, instead, recognize them as human beings who did the best they could with the tools they had.

Science is emphatic when it states that disciplinary approaches such as isolation (*time-outs* or thinking chairs), as well as shouting, humiliation, or threats, are not effective in the long term and also cause pain, fear, and stress in children, while keeping the child's brain in a state of hypervigilance because, as we have already seen, the amygdala becomes overexcited when it perceives the environment as threatening. Remember that threat does not only refer to situations in which our life is in imminent danger, such as being in the middle of a war. The feeling of danger is also perceived by our emotional brain when someone yells at us, humiliates us, looks at us harshly, ignores us, or points a finger at us, and this causes our amygdala to activate as if a snake were about to bite us.

I want you to imagine that you are walking through an open field and suddenly a wild dog appears in front of you. At that moment, your entire survival mechanism is activated and, as we have already seen, your amygdala and hypothalamus spring into action, immediately sending a signal to your pituitary gland, which in turn sends another signal to your adrenal gland with an alert message that would sound something like this: "Alert, alert, we need stress hormones, adrenaline, cortisol; we are in imminent danger."

All this work carried out by your brain causes your heart to start beating much harder and faster and your pupils to dilate. Your airways open up to leave you equipped and ready both to fight the dog and to flee from that place. As you can see, this response is wonderful and, above all, very adaptive when you are faced with a wild dog that intends to attack you. But what happens when we talk about a child, whose brain is still developing, who is vulnerable, and who is 100% dependent on their caregivers? That same alert and survival system is activated when they perceive that the person who walks through the door every evening and whom they call mom or dad creates the same fear in them that the wild dog creates in you and me. That same alert and survival system for imminent danger is repeatedly activated, leaving the child in a state of constant amygdala hyperarousal, known as amygdaloid hyperarousal. Therefore, the function of their amygdala, which is to keep them safe, goes from fulfilling an adaptive function, because it prepares them to protect themselves, to harming their mental health, because it remains activated and excited even after the danger has passed.

LeDoux has studied the role played by the amygdala in childhood and has reached a conclusion that seems to support one of the fundamental principles of psychoanalytic thinking, namely that the interaction of encounters and disagreements between the child and their caregivers during the early years of life constitutes genuine emotional learning. In LeDoux's view, this emotional learning is so powerful and so difficult for adults to understand because it is engraved in the amygdala with the rough, nonverbal imprint of emotional life."[5]

From a physiological and neurological point of view, when physical punishment is used, the areas of the emotional brain that we have already mentioned are activated because the brain perceives physical pain as a threat.

Imagine you are walking along the sidewalk on your way home when suddenly a thief appears with the intention of harming you. At that moment, the oldest part of your brain will go into what we call "alert mode" and you will try to flee, fight, or surrender. You see a police car approaching, and your own survival instinct pushes you to ask for help. The thief flees, and you finally receive the help you desperately needed at that moment. That police officer has been your calm in the midst of the storm.

Now imagine a child standing in front of his father, who threatens him with a slipper, a belt, or his own hand. Exactly the same thing happens as happened to you with the thief and with the example of the wild dog; the oldest part of his brain goes on alert and the same circuits in his brain will push him to seek help, to seek refuge. The paradoxical thing about this scene with the child is that, unlike the adult who found support in the police officer, the child finds that in his case, his own father, who should be a source of protection, becomes at the same time a source of terror. This confusion is what the great Daniel Siegel, referring to Mary Main, called an "insoluble biological paradox."

> "On the one hand, we are all born with the instinct to turn to our caregivers for protection when we are hurt or scared. However, if caregivers are also the source of pain and fear, if the parent has caused the child to feel terror because of something they have done, the situation can be very confusing for the child's brain, as it creates an unsolvable paradox."[6]

Therefore, if you are still wondering whether physical punishment can cause traumatic injury, my answer is yes. Let's remember that trauma alters a person's ability to feel safe with another person, given that their survival system is hyper-excited. So, if the person causing this insoluble fear in the child is their own caregiver, the underlying roots of development for secure attachment are broken.

Since at this point a thought may arise that sounds like "I was beaten and I wasn't traumatized," I want to conclude this section with one last statement.

Bessel van der Kolk mentions that trauma causes a fundamental reorganization of how the mind and brain handle perceptions. It changes not only how and what we think, but also our very ability to think.[7] In other words, much of the discourse of those who defend or may once have justified punishment, spanking, ignoring, or humiliating children is based both on their narrative and on the way they relate to their children. When these adults were children, they probably did not have a close experience of good treatment against which to compare their own experience. As a result, what they perceived as normal—abuse—was, in fact, an, undeserved, and harmful.

Growing up in an environment where abuse was normal and recurrent on a daily basis can give children the feeling of being alone, which is enough to put them on high alert and cause them to continue living that way into adulthood. Many of these children, now adults, may be struggling in life without yet realizing that much of their behavior patterns manifest traumatic responses, such as justifying abuse, precisely because they are traumatized.

The belief that "I was hit and I wasn't traumatized" is actually a response to trauma. If today, as adults, we continue to perpetuate this narrative in the way we relate to our children, what we are really showing is a traumatic wound.

This series of events emphasizes that every adult, with or without children, has a responsibility to know and understand, even if only minimally, what conscious and assertive parenting based on mutual respect consists of and how its presence or absence generates short- and long-term consequences in the lives of our children, including, of course, their mental health.

6.3 What makes an experience traumatic?

A child is not traumatized because they cry, get frustrated, or feel sad. A child is traumatized because they are left alone to deal with their fear, anger, or sadness.

When we talk about psychological trauma, we look beyond the event itself, which is of course fundamental. What happens around that experience—the discourse that the surrounding context creates about it—is what will largely determine whether the child is encourages to talk about what happened in order to heal or push to silence the experience under the belief that silence also heals: "time heals everything," "it's not that big of a deal," and "let's wipe the slate clean." Let us remember: what is traumatic is not only what happened, but also what was silenced, what was missing, and what was left unsaid.

No child will learn anything in life by being left alone in their pain. So, raise a red flag if, while raising your children, you hear:

- "Let them learn to defend themselves, you won't be there for them forever."
- "Let her cry. If you pay attention to her, she'll start manipulating you with her crying."
- "Those are crocodile tears to manipulate you."

The ability to overcome obstacles is learned in the company of *someone* who supports us emotionally, and the result of that support, that embrace, that "I'm here for you" is what we know as "resilience."

> Let's remember this: going through pain, anger, frustration, or sadness in the midst of loneliness makes our pain completely unmanageable.

The misconception that we learn to get through difficult situations alone, without any support, is, I believe, rooted in the core of trauma. Perhaps we have learned that asking for help or needing *someone else* to connect with is synonymous with weakness. But the truth is that our deepest and most natural impulses are toward connection with others. Therefore, it is not their sadness, anger, fear, or frustration that traumatizes our children, but rather the absence of a significant caregiver who provides comfort, support, empathy, and validation of their experience. The lack of emotional support is in itself another traumatic situation for the child. Therefore, learning to communicate with our children, including listening to them empathically, is a fundamental task as we educate them for life.

Assertive, loving, or cooperative communication encourages secure attachment while caring for our children's mental health and fostering trusts in the relationship. Scholars call this "contingent communication." The child sends a signal (fear, anger, sadness, or frustration), the adult perceives it, understands it, and responds to it by meeting the corresponding need (hunger, sleep, feeling seen, play, or connection). In response, the child is able to return to an optimal emotional state.

From the beginning of their existence, children need cooperative communication in order to mature properly. When a baby smiles and makes soft sounds, parents respond affectionately, smiling back, imitating their sounds, and then allowing the little one to respond again. This initiates a dialogue that conveys to the baby the message that their parents see them, listen to them, and reflect back an image of themselves that will be very valuable in helping them to see and value themselves. In short, parents are saying that they love their child just as they are."[8]

Imagine you are 3 years old and walking to the park with your mother. Suddenly, you see a very large dog approaching, and when it reaches you, it barks. You get scared and start crying, filled with anxiety. Your mother, who is doing everything she can to stop you from crying, says, "It's okay, it was just a bark." Seeing that you won't stop crying, she tries to comfort you by saying, "Look, here's some ice cream; eat it to get over your fright." This doesn't calm you down either, so your mother, tired, says, "Either you stop crying or we're leaving the park immediately."

Although your mother's real intention at that moment was for you to cope with the situation and come out on top, she wasn't really tuning in to your fear; she wasn't being contingent. You showed her that you needed support, and she responded with indifference. Your behavioral, emotional, and physiological response was to cry even more. Fear overwhelmed you because, among other things, you did not have the opportunity to express what you were feeling. Being so young, you did not have the words to do so, nor was there an adult who could act as an emotional translator to help you express what had happened to you by putting your feelings into words and, from there, accompany you to regulate yourself with their calm and presence, that is, to carry out the process of heteroregulation.

Every time you go to the park, you see the same dog and even other dogs, and you feel the same fear, anxiety, and desire to run away, while your mother's hand squeezes you tightly and she says again, "You know, if you start crying, we'll go home and that will be the end of the park."

Now you're an adult, and when you see a dog, you feel the same way you did when you were a child, even though you know rationally that the dog won't hurt you.

When we are children, our earliest memories are engraved in our implicit memory; that is, they are memories that are unconsciously recorded in our bodies in the form of bodily sensations. They do not have an orderly, coherent, and complete narrative, but they are charged with emotional content. Thus, when an implicit memory is activated in the here and now, it feels as if something from the past is happening in the present; we feel it viscerally in our body. That is why, when a child or any human being has an experience that impacts them emotionally, they need someone else to listen to them, legitimize them, and validate their feelings so that, from there, they can give meaning to the experience they have had. Therefore, I repeat what I said at the beginning: what makes an experience traumatic is not only what happened, but also what was missing, what was silenced, and what was not narrated.

Richard Erskine, clinical psychologist and psychoanalyst, states that "it is not trauma that destroys the human psyche, but the absence of a relationship during the time when a traumatic event occurs or immediately afterwards."

I must conclude by saying that contingent communication, in which, the child feels safe and secure because there is an adult interacting with them and responding to their needs, especially in the midst of experiences that impact them emotionally, largely determines the neural structures that will serve as the basis for their sense of "I am a loved and capable person," that is, for their sense of self. Daniel Siegel describes it this way: when we send out a signal, our brain remains receptive to the responses that other people may give to that signal. The responses we receive in this way end up being included in the neural maps that constitute our core sense of self. In this way, the brain generates a neural representation of that self that is dependent on others and ends up becoming a central element of our sense of identity.[9] In other words, when a child perceives that their parents consistently respond when they need them, the child not only feels comfortable, understood, loved, and valued by their caregiver, but also grows up with the feeling that they are not alone in the world, because they are connected to someone trustworthy who is helping them develop coherent, complete, integrated, and effective understanding of themselves and of the situations they experience.

So, returning to the example of the girl who was frightened by the dog, what would have been an appropriate response? We will examine this in the following section.

6.4 The four elements of contingent communication

It takes more than words to support our children when they are experiencing intense emotions: having managed to put together that puzzle that was so difficult for them, feeling frustrated because their fever ruined their weekend outing, feeling deeply saddened by the death of a loved one or their lifelong pet. All of these situations that could overwhelm our children emotionally require our presence, empathy, and contingent communication; that is, we need to help them narrate what they have experienced so that they can integrate that experience in an optimal way.

We have already discussed how traumatic experiences and the rupture of the attachment bond affect a child's ability to learn to regulate their emotions. Providing the foundations for self-regulation from an early age by fostering secure attachment is essential for the mental health of the child and the adult they will become. We can learn to self-regulate; however, heteroregulation is a process that we need throughout our lives. At some point, we will need someone else to provide us with support, comfort, and understanding, regardless of our age. And all of this can be learned when we have received it primarily from our attachment figures. Therefore, in order to talk about self-regulation, we first need to talk about heteroregulation.

From heteroregulation to self-regulation

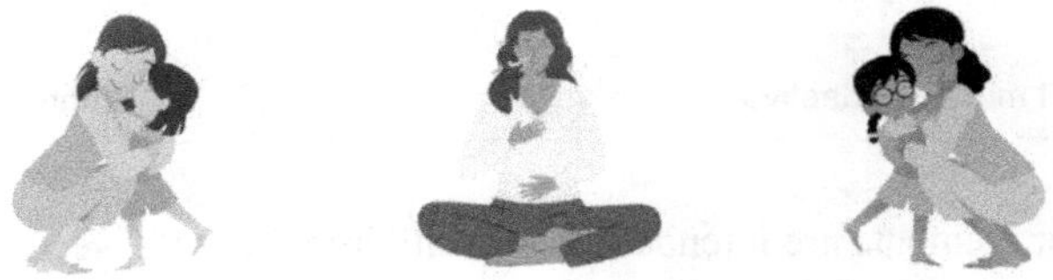

You teach me to regulate myself (heteroregulation) | I have learned to self-regulate | I can heteroregulate others

As we can see, contingent communication is associated with heteroregulation because without an emotional connection, there is no learning. If we do not convey compassion and understanding with our nonverbal language (right hemisphere), the narrative we offer our children through our words (left hemisphere) is not effective. We must integrate warmth, understanding, compassion, and unconditional acceptance with consistency, linearity, and discourse about what has happened; that is, we must integrate our right hemisphere (emotional brain) with our left hemisphere (rational brain).

If we already possess compassion, unconditional love, and empathetic and assertive nonverbal language, what are the precise words needed to ensure that the narrative our child internalizes is complete, coherent, effective, and comprehensive? How can we achieve this?

To make this easier to remember, focus on four elements when telling your child the story of an experience:[10]

- Body
- Cognitions
- Behavior
- Emotions

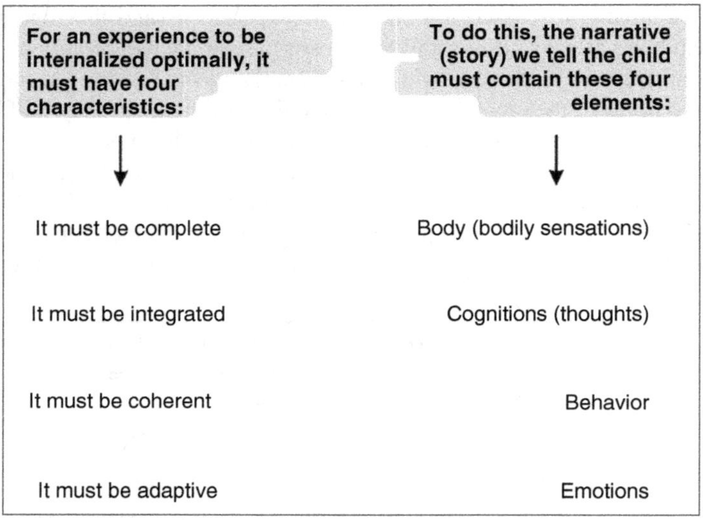

These four elements are intended to help children feel safe, secure, and empowered with the story we first tell them about what happened and then, later, they will tell themselves about what happened and how they experienced it, integrating what happened outside and how it impacted them inside. When you do this, you are helping your child regulate themselves through your heteroregulation.

Let's look at each of them in more detail.

6.4.1 Body

When we talk about the body, we are referring to bodily sensations. Remember that every experience has a bodily component. Make sure that the story you tell your child includes this aspect, and to do so, you could use words such as *observe, perceive, and notice.*

Here are some of them:

- Sweating
- Rapid heartbeat
- Rapid breathing
- Cold hands
- Stomach ache
- Dizziness
- Lump in the throat
- Shaking hands, legs, or whole body
- Chest pressure
- Hot face

6.4.2 *Cognitions*

Cognitions are the thoughts or ideas that come to mind when we are going through that specific situation. The two words we will use to include this element in the story are *think* or *believe.* Here are some examples of cognitions:

- "... that's why you believed the dog was going to bite you..."
- "... that's why you think you won't be able to pass the exam, because..."
- "Sometimes you may come to believe that it's not possible because..."
- "...and you think we should stay longer in the park to..."

6.4.3 *Behavior*

When we talk about behavior, we are referring to what we do or the actions that are triggered by a specific situation: shouting, crying, biting, hitting, etc. Therefore, the word we usually use in the story we tell our children is related to the word "do" and other verbs that express what the child has done as a result of that situation. It is usually preceded by the phrase "... that's why":

- "... that's why you hit your cousin."
- "...that's why you started crying."
- "...that's why you ran away."
- "...that's why you screamed for help."

6.4.4 *Emotions*

This point is often complicated when we include it in the narrative or story we give our children, because we lack emotional vocabulary. We have learned that we feel *good* or *bad.* And in those two phrases that do not express an emotional correlate, we tend to summarize our entire internal experience, generating an incoherent, incomplete, ineffective, and disintegrated narrative.

To include emotions in the narrative we give our children, we use the word "feel." At this point, I recommend referring to the seven basic emotions that all human beings feel, regardless of our beliefs, culture, or place of birth:

- Love
- Joy
- Curiosity
- Fear
- Anger
- Sadness
- Shame

If you want to enrich your emotional vocabulary, I also highly recommend the book *Emocionario*[11] and the children's story by Mercedes Bermejo *Plantánimals. La emocipedia infantil.*[12]

In our next chapter, we will also address the topic of emotional intelligence. But first, let me show you what a story might sound like with the four elements that a narrative must contain in order to be complete, integrated, coherent, and adaptive:

"Honey, your heart is racing and your hands are cold; you're scared because the dog got too close to us, right? When you heard it bark loudly, you thought it was going to bite you, so you screamed and started crying. I'm here with you, you're safe, you're secure."

Notes

1 Aznárez, B. (2021). *El trauma psíquico es de todos. Rompe el silencio.* Edición: www.triunfacontulibro.com.

2 Van der Kolk, B. (2017), *El cuerpo lleva la cuenta. Cerebro, mente y cuerpo en la superación del trauma.* Barcelona: Eleftheria.

3 Van der Kolk, B. (2017), *El cuerpo lleva la cuenta. Cerebro, mente y cuerpo en la superación del trauma.* Barcelona: Eleftheria.

4 Siegel, D. J., and Bryson, T. P. (2019). *Disciplina sin lágrimas Una guía imprescindible para orientar y alimentar el desarrollo mental de tu hijo.* Barcelona: Penguin Random House Grupo Editorial.

5 Goleman, D. (1996). *Inteligencia Emocional.* Barcelona: Editorial Kairós.

6 Siegel, D. J., and Bryson, T. P. (2019). *Disciplina sin lágrimas Una guía imprescindible para orientar y alimentar el desarrollo mental de tu hijo.* Barcelona: Penguin Random House Grupo Editorial.

7 Van der Kolk, B. (2017), *El cuerpo lleva la cuenta. Cerebro, mente y cuerpo en la superación del trauma.* Barcelona: Eleftheria.

8 Hartzell, M., and Siegel, D. (2019), *Ser padres conscientes.* Barcelona: Ediciones La Llave.

9 Hartzell, M., and Siegel, D. (2019), *Ser padres conscientes.* Barcelona: Ediciones La Llave.

10 These four elements are based on the psychotherapeutic intervention model developed by Begoña Aznárez and José Luis Marín, presidents of the Spanish Association of Psychosomatic Medicine and Psychotherapy.

11 Núñez, C., and Valcárcel, R. (2013). *Emocionario. Di lo que sientes.* Madrid: Palabras Aladas.

12 Bermejo, M. (2019). *Plantánimals. La emocipedia infantil.* Barcelona: Editorial Marcombo.

Chapter 7

Emotions, the great unknowns

The more open we are to our own feelings, the better we can read those of others.
(Daniel Goleman)

As we have seen so far, emotions are at the root of what we know as *internal experience.* There is no experience that does not contain emotional content: when our team wins the game, we feel intense joy; when we say goodbye to someone we love so much, we feel sadness; when we are in the park and see a child hitting our son and his father does not even flinch, we may feel anger. When we are at home and suddenly hear an unexpected noise that makes us jump, we may feel fear. Our experiences are endowed with somatosensory, cognitive, behavioral, and, of course, emotional content.

I believe that, before continuing, it is necessary to begin by defining what an emotion is, and to do so, we return to the Royal Spanish Academy (RAE), which defines emotion as an "intense and temporary change in mood, pleasant or painful, accompanied by a certain somatic commotion."

Although this definition is quite general, it emphasizes an important point, which is that emotion is intense and fleeting. It is precisely these two aspects that differentiate emotions from feelings. While a basic emotion such as fear can be experienced intensely and fleetingly, a feeling such as helplessness can linger over time. What is the difference between the two? While fear can be intense and momentary, helplessness is the sum of fear plus a cognition or belief. "I won't be able to do it."

EMOTION: Intense and fleeting reaction
FEELING: Basic emotion + belief

Similarly, when we talk about fear and anxiety, we can differentiate between them in that fear would be an intense and momentary reaction to a real or objective danger, while anxiety would be the sum of fear plus one or more cognitions ("this is bigger than me"); which generates excessive concern about real situations and, above all, about events that have not yet occurred.

DOI: 10.4324/9781003784487-7

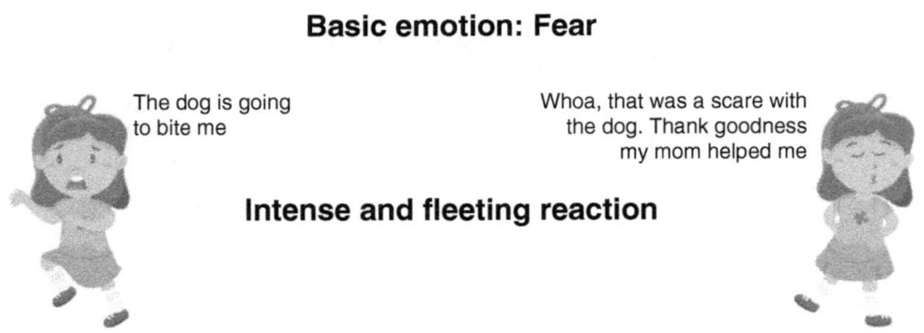

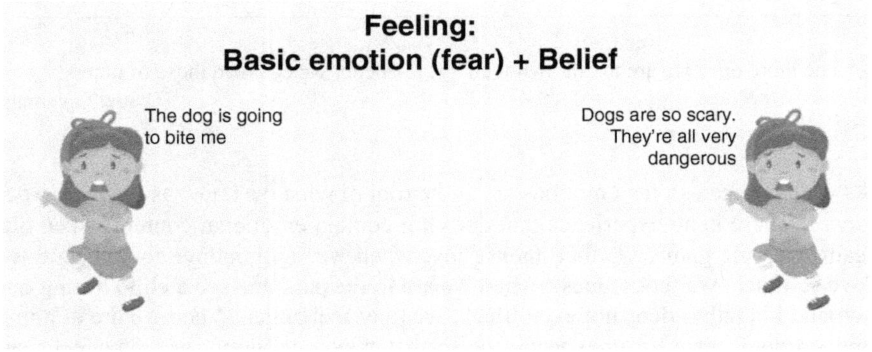

In the case of children who are constantly anxious, we can observe this in intrusive thoughts or cognitive distortions when faced with school exams ("I'm going to forget everything again during the exam and I'm going to fail"), relationships with their friends ("nobody likes me because I'm a foreigner") or the physical health of their family, mainly their parents; For example, children with panic attacks at the thought that their mother could die at any moment. All of these situations can significantly interfere with a child's normal daily activities. Later on, we will learn how we can help them to promote balance and resilience.

7.1 All emotions "have their talent": there are no good or bad emotions

Emotions are neither good nor bad; they are neither negative nor positive: emotions are adaptive and functional. We need them to live, to defend ourselves, to bond with others, to separate ourselves from others. They are a great gift that we have been given, and ignoring or disregarding them has given them a very bad reputation.

All basic emotions have their talent: they inform us of danger and injustice; they help us overcome obstacles and work through grief; they give us courage and move us toward connection and, if necessary, toward distancing ourselves.

Daniel Goleman says in his well-known *bestseller*[1] that "all emotions are, in essence, impulses that drive us to act." Hence, the etymological root of the word *emotion* comes from the Latin verb *movere*, which means "to move," plus the prefix e, which means something like "movement toward"; that is, in every emotion there is an implicit tendency toward action.

In child psychology, we have learned that children are psychocorporal, which means that they express their emotions through their bodies. That is why, when they feel joy, they jump; when they are angry, they may bite, scream, or hit; when they feel ashamed, they may try to hide between our legs; and when they are afraid, they may scream disproportionately for help. Helping them integrate their emotional and physical worlds through our interpretation, legitimization, and validation is an important task that every caregiver must carry out so that all that emotional baggage is not ignored and thus dissociated, but rather can be seen and addressed with the appropriate affection. As Daniel Siegel would say, our job as caregivers is to help our children integrate their right (emotional) hemisphere with their left (rational) hemisphere.

This helps ensure that their experiences and the memories of them are as well integrated and organized as possible, as we saw in Chapter 3.

7.2 Basic emotions and the two major psychobiological systems: approach and defense

We have just explained that there are no good or bad, positive or negative emotions, but rather that they are all functional and adaptive. In turn, when emotions are intense and fleeting, we are referring exclusively to basic emotions, since, as we explained, if they remain over time, then they cease to be a basic emotion and become a feeling.

Basic emotions have been studied for many years; some group them into the five best known: love, fear, joy, sadness, and anger. The following list brings these five emotions together for easy reference:

Love

Fear

Joy

Sadness

Anger

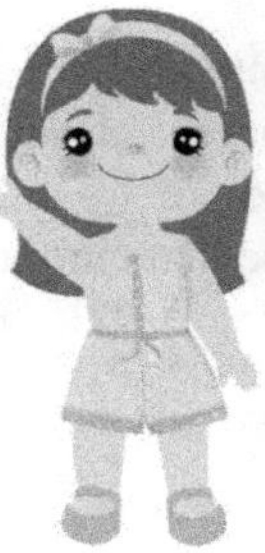

However, I would like to share with you two more emotions on this list of basic emotions that I added during my training as a psychotherapist. These emotions are curiosity and shame. I should mention that many studies and experts consider shame to be a social emotion, like guilt and pride, rather than a basic emotion, because, unlike the other emotions we have already mentioned, it does not appear until around the age of three, when there has been greater brain maturation in some specific areas, which in turn allows for more complex processes, such as the mental imagination of situations.

Okay, now that we have clarified the difference between an emotion and a feeling and what the so-called basic emotions are, I want us to understand a little more about their adaptive function.

Pierre Janet was a French psychologist, neurologist, and philosopher who introduced the concept of *the psychobiological approach system and psychobiological defense system* to explain the adaptive function of emotions. The former refers to our need to bond with others, and the latter has the function of helping us keep our distance from stimuli (objects, people, or situations) that we find threatening. Therefore, depending on whether we perceive a stimulus as dangerous or friendly, we will respond with one emotion or another, and depending on the characteristics of that stimulus and our emotional response, we will place that basic emotion in one of these two systems.

If a child perceives that, in the midst of a tantrum, their mother gets down to their level, looks at them compassionately, and tries to help them regulate their anger, the child will perceive their mother as a source of comfort. This will activate their psychobiological approach system and cause the anger response to gradually lose intensity. By contrast, if that same child sees their mother approaching in the midst of the tantrum with a slipper raised to hit them and a finger pointed at them, the child will perceive her as a threat.

Their psychobiological defense system will then be activated, and they will respond mainly with fear, since this emotion is, as Begoña Aznárez says, "the mother of all emotions." A child's greatest fear, albeit unconscious, is the fear of abandonment, of becoming detached from their primary attachment figures. Therefore, if that child, in the midst of his anger, has to conclude that he is a "bad child" rather than recognize that his father or mother has made a mistake, he will do so, because in childhood, for survival, attachment takes precedence over everything else.

"Approach and defense systems are like earth, water, and light. They play a crucial role in the development of our personality and explain, in my opinion, eighty percent or more of who we are and what we do."[2] According to these two major systems and the impulse that emotion drives us toward, we would have the following outline:

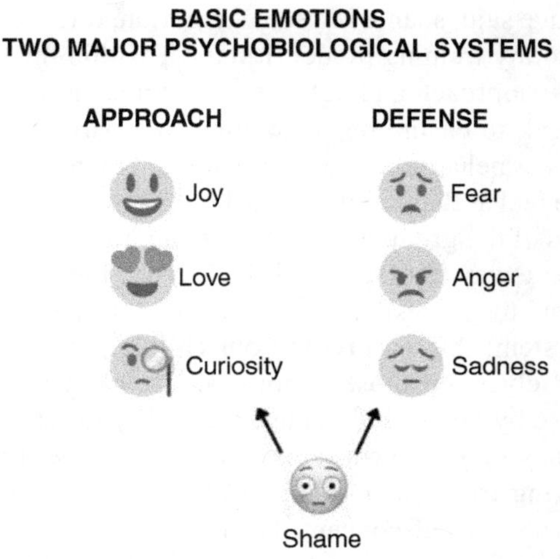

Approach emotions: joy, love, and curiosity are three emotions that motivate us to connect with stimuli that invite us to do so. A mother's love for her baby moves her to care for, feed, and protect it, and in turn, the child perceives her care and generates that connection and bond. A father's joy when he sees his daughter walk for the first time moves him to hug her, encourage her, and in turn, her response becomes a mobilizer of the girl's bond with her caregiver. Curiosity is the emotion that leads children to take an interest in their surroundings, not only in terms of what they discover cognitively through new flavors, smells, textures, etc., but also in terms of their own species: their parents, close relatives and, later on, classmates, cultures, or countries.

Defensive emotions: fear, anger, and sadness drive us toward disengagement, rejection, and the need to distance ourselves. In fact, we can observe the sequence of these three emotions in the order in which I present them to you. Let me give you an example. When a girl is at school and sees that she has failed her math exam, she may initially feel fear about the consequences that her result may have at home. Immediately afterwards, she may need to feel anger in order to seek justice and, weathering her emotional storm, she may approach her teacher and tell him that, because of a "simple 2 she missed in the second exercise, it is not fair that she should fail the whole exam." Or she may not go to her teacher at all, but instead go to her classmate to say that the teacher is very unfair and seems to have something against her. After feeling fear and anger, sadness arises and the need to connect with it in order to process the grief that comes with things not turning out as expected. Yes, losing is inherent to being alive, and we lose every day: we lose objects, people, ideals, beliefs, expectations, desires.

Shame: as we have said, shame is a social emotion, often mislabeled as "negative." According to my training model, I place it within the two major psychobiological systems: approach and defense. Sometimes it drives us to bond with others when we seek to ensure our belonging to a particular group and notice that certain aspects or behaviors of ours could jeopardize our acceptance by others. The shame we feel at that moment "pushes" us to act in accordance with the standards or norms of the group we want to belong to, "mortgaging" our desires and interests in some way in order to "fit in." Hence the importance of working on it and its "talent" to give voice to its adaptive function from the psychobiological defense system; that is, inviting our children to reflect, and doing this same exercise ourselves, on those actions we are carrying out or avoiding in order to be accepted by others and to have the ability to set assertive boundaries which, although they may also cause us shame at first, will be necessary when what I am perceiving from outside is putting my integrity as a person at risk. Shame is in tune with our self-concept. The more dignified, loved, accepted, and valuable our children feel in their relationship with us, the greater their ability to set assertive boundaries with others, even if this means distancing themselves at times.

7.2.1 *Shame*

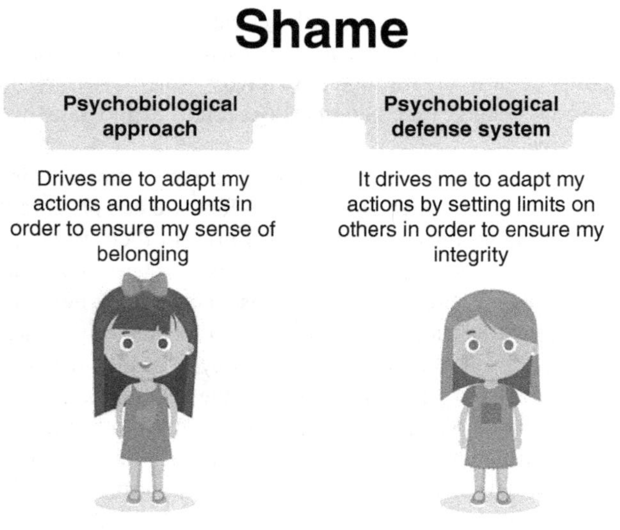
Shame
Psychobiological approach
Drives me to adapt my actions and thoughts in order to ensure my sense of belonging
Psychobiological defense system
It drives me to adapt my actions by setting limits on others in order to ensure my integrity

7.3 Emotions explained to adults and children

So far, we have seen that basic emotions motivate us, are functional, help us adapt to situations, and even enable us to set assertive boundaries when our personal integrity is at risk or when, on the contrary, we want to belong.

Emotions are far from being good or bad, positive or negative, as they have been mislabeled for so long. But then, how do we explain to our children that even if they feel angry, they should not hurt others?

I think that's where we need to focus, on the fact that what we feel is one thing and what we do with those feelings is another. That's what can lead to the mistaken belief that it's wrong to feel, that emotions are bad, and you can teach your child the difference between their emotions and their behavior.

Anger is one of the emotions that causes us the most discomfort and conflict when we see it on the surface in our children. I usually explain to my children the difference between feeling angry and what we do with that anger in the following way:

Imagine that anger is like a dragon inside us. When someone has done something you don't like or things haven't turned out the way you expected, you feel angry and you may feel that anger like a ball of fire burning inside you (physical sensation). If, in the midst of your anger, you start shaking the dragon inside you, shouting at it, swearing at it, or hitting it, the dragon will breathe fire that will come out through your mouth, hurting you and hurting others.

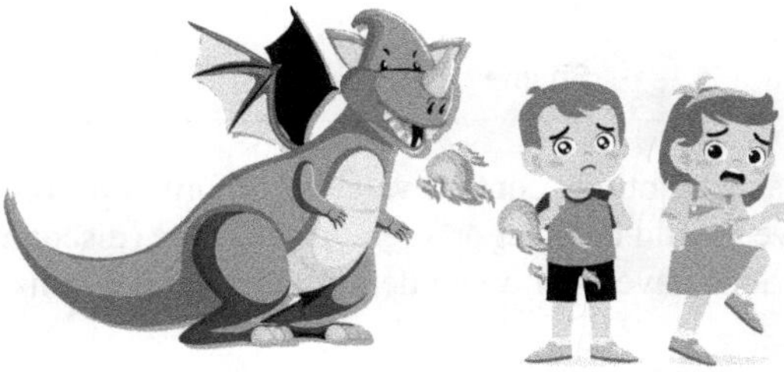

But if, in the midst of your anger, you gently approach the dragon, you will also feel that ball of fire burning inside you (physical sensation), and at the same time you will be able to breathe so that little by little that fire will decrease in intensity and will not come out and hurt others, but neither will it remain inside and hurt you. To do this, we can breathe like horses. This means that we take air in through our nose and release it through our mouth, moving our lips like horses. Each time we take in air and release it, we gradually extinguish the intensity of the fire. Once its intensity is reduced, we can talk about what happened.

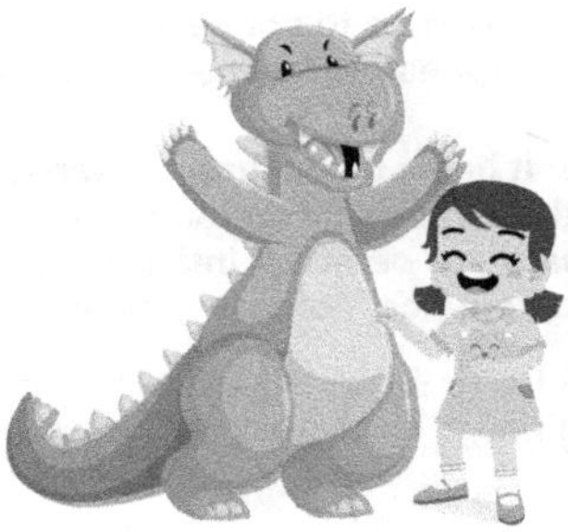

Anger is an emotion that mobilizes us "outwardly"; just as joy, love, curiosity, and shame (when seeking to disengage) make us feel physically and mentally vigorous, while fear, sadness, and often shame (when seeking to engage) mobilize us "inwardly," we may end up feeling physically and mentally depleted, with very few resources, possibilities, and options.

They drive us outward	They drive us inward
Anger	Fear
Joy	Sadness
Curiosity	Shame
Love	
Shame	

However, all basic emotions contain valuable information for our survival that tells us whether we should connect or keep our distance (disconnect). I like to say that all basic emotions have their own talent. Let me explain this in more detail.

ALL EMOTIONS HAVE THEIR OWN TALENT

Anger: It helps us overcome obstacles and seek justice and fairness.

Joy: It helps us by lifting our spirits and motivating us to build and maintain relationships.

Curiosity: Helps us maintain the desire to explore learn, step outside our comfort zone, and grow in all areas.

Love: It drives us to connect with others and is largely responsible for the survival of the species.

Shame: It helps us ensure our sense of belonging (from the "approach" perspective) and also safeguard our personal integrity (from the psychobiological defense system).

Fear: It helps us anticipate threats and seek protection.

Sadness: It helps us remain still, at rest, and inactive so we can process our losses and reintegrate.

7.4 Integrating emotion and behavior with the MAC method

In Chapter 3, we talked about the importance of integrating both hemispheres to connect emotionally with our children (right hemisphere), while redirecting their behavior (left hemisphere).

Imagine that your 7-year-old son comes into your room after you have finally managed to get him to fall asleep, and says to you:

"I'm afraid that one day we'll all go out and I'll get lost and never see you again." You, who still don't understand where he got that idea from and who are just trying to finish the work you couldn't do during the day, reply: "Don't think about things like that, nothing's going to happen. Go to sleep; it's late and I'm tired." Your son insists and replies: "I'm scared and I don't want to go to my room to sleep alone."

There isn't a single session or workshop where I don't hear a parent tell me that they are tired of their children's excuses or complaints about meaningless things. When we experience situations similar to the example, it is often frustrating because we feel that we have given our all during the day and that the little space we have is suddenly interrupted for reasons that, in our opinion, sound illogical. "Milena is no longer two years old (she is seven, eight, nine), and she can't possibly continue to think and behave like a little girl." The truth is that, although it may sound illogical to us, there are moments, even many moments, in our child's speech when they are actually going through "emotional turmoil" coming from their right hemisphere, which makes it impossible for the logical and coherent explanations of the left hemisphere to bring peace to their soul. In fact, what usually happens is that we respond as the mother in the example did, with logical but ultimately ineffective explanations:

"Since you were born, when has there been an earthquake? Never!";

"You're thinking that because you're in front of the screen," "What you want is for me to go to bed with you, and you don't realize that I've been putting off my own things all day to be with you." These responses, based on rational explanations from the left hemisphere, in the face of the emotional barrage from our children's right hemisphere, create a gap between them and us. When one hemisphere dominates, the other "shuts down" and becomes inactive. Therefore, when we focus on responding from our logic at times when they are in the midst of an emotional avalanche, our children will feel more misunderstood and less receptive to our words. In other words, when your child is in the midst of an "emotional hijacking," your logical explanations are bound to fail.

So, instead of starting a power struggle, it would be more effective to first connect with their emotional world in the right hemisphere and then access their left hemisphere with logical explanations focused on the here and now. This is what we call "emotional connection," although I prefer to call it "emotional attunement": putting ourselves on the same emotional wavelength as our child at that moment. However, put like that, it may sound abstract; we need to know "how to do it," how to put it into practice in those moments. I call this the "MAC method."

THE MAC METHOD

Modeling

Acompany

Channel

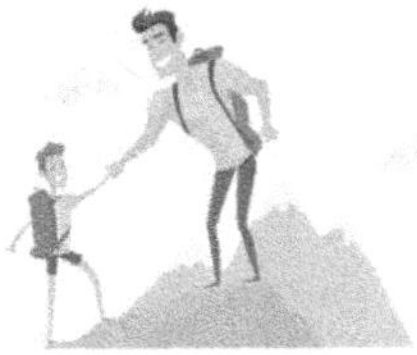

Modeling: our Western society constantly turns to reason and words to solve problems. This may be effective with an adult, but it is counterproductive with a child whose brain is still maturing. Modeling means reflecting the emotional state we want to see in our children in those moments of chaos. Modeling does not mean stopping feeling or remaining calm at all times. It is impossible to stop feeling overwhelmed, angry, afraid, or frustrated when our child is in the middle of a tantrum, an anxiety attack, or an emotional outburst.

Modeling has to do with:

- Validating our own emotional state (it is valid for me to feel frustrated by this situation; I am not a bad mother for feeling this way right now).
- Naming what we feel (anger, fear, tiredness, etc.).
- Taking charge of my emotional world: breathing techniques, counting to ten, drinking water, splashing cold water on your face, looking at your height and how tall and big you are compared to your little one, or looking at the size of their hands and feet in those moments also helps us remember that they are just a child who needs us deeply.

When our child is in the midst of an "emotional hijack" and we become overwhelmed in the same way or even worse, what is happening is what is known as "emotional contagion," that is, through mirror neurons, our own nervous system is activated and reflects the same state of arousal as our child's nervous system. The same physical sensations you feel at that moment, such as rapid heartbeat, sweating, tightness in the chest, or cold hands, are the sensations your child is feeling too.

Therefore, only when we are able to validate, attend to, and sustain our own emotional world will we be prepared to consistently project the emotional state we want to see in our children. When faced with the emotional outbursts of others, we must first attend to our own internal state so that we can reflect, as if in a mirror, the optimal emotional state we want to see in them. Only then will your calmness be their calmness.

Making a conscious decision to stand in front of my child as if I were a mirror, with the most genuine intention of helping them, means putting ourselves at their level, establishing eye contact and, if they allow us, maintaining physical contact (a hug, a kiss, our hands on their hands…). Most of the time, there is no need to say anything during those moments, just to be available and present.

Accompany: this has to do with being responsive and contingent to the emotional need that our child expresses at that moment, no matter how absurd their behavior may seem to us. When your 8-year-old tells you that he hates his brother, instead of telling him right then and there that you don't use those words in your house, appeal to his right brain by saying something like, "Wow, you seem really angry. Tell me more," or, if you are like the mother in the example we started with, connect with their right brain by speaking from your own experience: "I remember when I was little, I was also afraid that I or someone I loved very much was in danger, and thoughts came to mind that made me feel sad; so sometimes they made me cry even though those things didn't happen."

When I say this, parents often ask me whether it is actually effective or whether they are simply giving in to their children's manipulation. But assertive parenting is not about avoiding limits or doing whatever our children want. It is about connecting before correcting and setting limits from a calm, regulated state.

Knowing how the brain works is revealing; it's like the missing piece of the puzzle that helps us understand how our children think, feel, and behave. Understanding this helps us get our children to cooperate much more readily, making those moments when things don't go as expected less complicated.

Channeling: according to the RAE, channeling means "to regulate the course or flow of a stream." And I love to bring up this definition to explain what I want to convey to you at this point. When we talk about emotional overflow, we can bring to mind the image of an overflowing river, in which, when the right brain takes control, it overwhelms our children and us with the chaos of emotions, and when the left brain takes control, it overwhelms us with the inflexibility of arguments and logic. Therefore, channeling has to do with integrating our hemispheres, validating and connecting with the emotional chaos that is fostered in the right brain and then giving way to the words and logic of the left hemisphere. Emotions are channeled through connection, and words are channeled when we intentionally choose empathy so that our child feels understood, heard, and with their emotional world translated or, as Siegel says, so that the child "feels felt." The integration of the two hemispheres through the channeling of emotions and logic would be what I call "empathic logic"; that is, intentionally chosen words that have first passed through the filter of emotion, ceasing to be cold words and becoming heartfelt words. Continuing with the example we started with, after modeling our child's emotional state and accompanying them, being responsive and contingent to their emotional needs, we could appeal to their left hemisphere by telling them what we could do if something like that were to happen.

Nothing calms our nervous system more, after being comforted, than having clear and accurate information about what to do in times of stress and distress. And this, in turn, is a way to prevent things from getting worse. This happened to us at home, and we saw it as an opportunity to empower our children in case it happened again. The next day, we drew up an action plan in case this happened and divided it into four steps:

- Stay where you are. Avoid running around.
- From where you are, see if you can spot your father or mother, a relative, or someone in authority (police officer, security guard, firefighter). If you don't see any of these people, look for a mother with children like you and say:
- "Help me, I'm lost."
- If you don't see any family members or mothers with children, then it's time to shout loudly, "Help, I'm lost." And right then, adults will come to your rescue.
- Always keep in mind that I do everything I can to find you and keep you safe and secure.

Channeling emotions and logic to integrate our children's brains is not something that works like a magic wand. We cannot forget that our children are unique and there are times when several factors may come together to create an emotional storm of such magnitude that it seems impossible to get through. Sometimes, it is enough just to be there; sometimes, it is enough just to model behavior. In many cases, waiting is the key, rather than saying anything, no matter how empathetic it may sound. Regardless of whether we wait or not, we must ensure that our children know that we are that safe haven they can turn to for refuge.

Notes

1 Goleman, D. (1996), *Inteligencia Emocional*. Barcelona: Editorial Kairós.
2 Aznárez, B. (2021), *El trauma psíquico es de todos. Rompe el silencio*. Edición: www.triunfacontulibro.com.

Chapter 8

Anxiety and mental health

> The role of "security" in life is so intuitive and relevant that it is striking that institutions do not take it into account. Perhaps our lack of knowledge of the function of safety may be due to the fact that we believe we know what safety means.
>
> (Stephen W. Porges)

Anxiety occupies a prominent place in clinical consultations, literature, and scientific research in the field of psychology. My intention, rather than addressing the different theoretical studies and scientific approaches that have been developed over the years, is to explain how anxiety affects your child, what causes it, and what you can do to help them, whether or not they develop an anxiety disorder.

Let us begin by looking at the concept of anxiety in the clinical setting.

We often confuse fear with anxiety. The truth is that fear, as we have already seen, is a basic adaptive and functional emotion that is usually intense, temporary, and expressed in the here and now. It arises as an emotional reaction to a present danger or to a stimulus perceived as dangerous; once that danger or stimulus has passed, the intensity of the emotion subsides. Anxiety, on the other hand, is a disproportionately intense reaction that initially arises from an emotion, fear, but is also associated with a limiting thought or belief ("I'll never be able to do it," "this is impossible," etc.).

"We are all going to die"), even when there is no objective evidence for this; that is, when nothing is happening to indicate that these beliefs are likely to occur.

We have all felt anxiety at some point in our lives, such as when facing a job interview, changing residence, or dealing with the death of a loved one. We might say that, in part, anxiety also has some value when it puts us on alert and prepares us to stay safe. The problem arises when it manifests itself for no apparent reason or when its intensity and duration are excessive. In these cases, we talk about anxiety disorders, which, according to the Diagnostic and Statistical Manual of Mental Disorders, must persist for at least 6 months. Among the most common are generalized anxiety disorder, specific phobia, social phobia, selective mutism, and agoraphobia.

DOI: 10.4324/9781003784487-8

Anxiety is a response to the anticipation of a future danger that is indefinable and unpredictable, with a cause that is vaguer and less understandable than fear. This response is experienced on a physical and behavioral level. Remember the four elements common to all experiences: body, cognition, behavior, and emotion.

8.1 Anxiety and the brain

I want to return to the brain again, but instead of explaining it based on its horizontal maturation (from right to left), as we saw in Chapter 3 and Chapter 7, let's imagine it as a two-story house. In other words, let's talk about vertical brain maturation (from bottom to top).

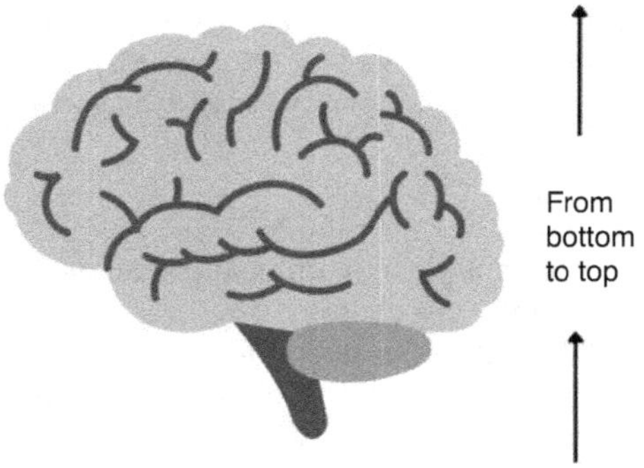

When a child is born, their lower brain, composed of, among other parts, the brain stem and the limbic system or emotional brain, is fully developed. This lower part of the brain, the brain stem, is responsible for basic and automatic functions such as breathing, blinking, sleep, and wakefulness. It is also responsible for innate reactions such as fight or flight and for defensive emotions such as anger and fear (limbic system). Our bodily sensations and instinctive behaviors derive from this lower part of the brain.

The higher brain is very different; it is much more complex and takes much longer to mature. Studies on the brain indicate that it matures between the ages of 25 and 30. Composed of the neocortex and the medial prefrontal cortex, it is responsible for thinking, imagination, and helping us make decisions, plan, manage our emotions and our bodily responses, and put ourselves in someone else's shoes; that is, it is responsible for sophisticated executive functions.

As with the case of the hemispheres, when the upper and lower brain are integrated, human beings function and behave better. Therefore, one of the most important tasks we can perform as caregivers is to help our children achieve this vertical integration because they cannot carry out this complex task on their own. There are basically two basic reasons for this. The first has to do, as we already mentioned, with the time it takes for the prefrontal cortex (upper brain) to develop. Understanding this is fundamental because, when you know that decision-making, empathy, anticipation, conflict resolution, as well as the ability to manage emotions and the impulses that drives us, are sophisticated functions of a mature brain, you understand that your young child does not have the ability to perform many tasks that you may have been demanding of them up to now because you were unaware of this fact about the brain; for example, they may not be able to learn on the first try, avoid becoming scared or angry about things that don't make sense to you, always put themselves in other people's shoes, or reflect altruistically on their problematic behavior and propose solutions for the situation. Knowing what you now know about the brain helps you set appropriate expectations according to your child's individual development.

The second reason why our children find it difficult to stay calm, manage their own fears on their own, react proportionately to stimuli that may seem harmless to us, and integrate their lower brain with their upper brain has to do with a part of their brain located in the limbic system called the "amygdala."

The amygdala, which actually consists of two amygdalae located above our brain stem near the limbic system and interconnected by a set of structures that give it an almond shape (in fact, *amygdala* comes from the Greek word meaning *almond*), is responsible for helping us process and express anger and fear in particular in a matter of milliseconds. Daniel Goleman, referring to LeDoux, calls it the "emotional sentinel" because of its role as the brain's "guard dog," keeping us alert to any possible signs that threaten our survival. It is the amygdala that causes us to act without stopping to think when we see our 2-year-old child near the pool trying to reach the rubber duck that has just fallen in. When you shout their name effusively, warning them that they are about to fall, and rush out to rescue them, almost losing your life in the process, remember that it is your amygdala that is doing everything possible to keep you and your loved ones safe. If the amygdala senses the slightest hint of danger, it can take complete control, inhibiting your higher brain and allowing you to act before you think.

This reaction is ideal when you or your child is facing a situation of imminent danger. However, reacting disproportionately and constantly when we are faced with situations that do not threaten our life or survival is not usually an adaptive response, and it is precisely in those moments that the amygdala, instead of helping us function by adapting to situations, can get us into trouble. Because there are situations in which, instead of acting before thinking, we need to think before acting so that we don't go through life lashing out at others and losing our composure. That state of control and balance is surely what you want for yourself and your children; that they can remain calm, especially in situations that have the potential to upset them, whether through anger or fear.

As we have seen throughout this book, your role as a caregiver is not to prevent every situation that overwhelms your child or to rescue them from it. Your role is to accompany them and, in a way, to "lend" them your mature prefrontal cortex, your words, and your capacity to reason. This helps them maintain balance in that moment and, through many hours and years of teaching and practice, gradually enables them to do so even when you are not there. You serve as a "ladder," helping them integrate what they feel in their lower brain with the calm and reflection of their higher brain.

This is not a question of one dominating the other, but rather of each contributing its "talent" to the emotional well-being of our children. In fact, one of the objectives is to teach them to make decisions with a sensible plan of action from their higher brain, while integrating the emotional and physical sensitivity that originates in their lower brain. Let's remember that when we educate, we do so for the moment, but above all, we do it for life.

8.2 Anxiety and the metaphor of the car

The basis of anxiety is a sense of insecurity. Not feeling safe or secure activates the defense mechanisms of our autonomic nervous system: fight, flight, freeze, or surrender.

Stephen W. Porges' polyvagal theory explains that feeling safe depends on the autonomic state and that signs of safety help to calm the autonomic nervous system.[1] When our nervous system is hyper- or hypoaroused, it affects our body and our ability to participate and relate to others.

Porges emphasizes the great importance of connecting and heteroregulating with others as the essence of our human biology. People need others in order to survive, and this imperative is even more relevant in childhood, as children consciously and unconsciously seek security in their caregivers. This state of security can only be achieved when you are their secure base, their life coach, and the harbor from which they feel safe to go out and explore the world and return to you when things outside become difficult. When your child is afraid or feels any other emotion, especially one arising from their biological defense system, your role is not to numb or distract them from what they are feeling, but to accompany them through their storm. Daniel Siegel, in line with polyvagal theory, calls this "help our children increase their window of tolerance." To explain this, he uses a metaphor that I think is very apt here.

The autonomic nervous system has two evolved branches. One is called the "sympathetic nervous system," and the other is the "parasympathetic nervous system." The first works like a car's accelerator; it injects us with the energy, movement, and emotional and physical vitality we need to carry out our tasks. It prepares our body by accelerating our heart rate and breathing, and by activating our muscles to get us going. The other branch does the opposite: it works like the brakes on a car, helping us to reduce our state of arousal, relaxing our muscles, allowing us to breathe much more slowly and bringing us back to calm. When adults and children perceive and feel that they are in a safe environment, our sympathetic and parasympathetic nervous systems work properly. In general, we tend to move through the day in this state of balance. However, when your 2-year-old spills milk on himself just before leaving the house and you feel tightness in your chest, a flushed face, and an intense desire to scream, you are experiencing increased sympathetic activity. By contrast, when you have just finished eating on a Sunday, you lie down on the sofa to watch TV, your eyelids feel heavy, and you can't stop yawning, you have increased parasympathetic activity.

When your child's sympathetic and parasympathetic nervous systems are in balance, they are said to be in their green zone or window of tolerance. They are able to ask you for the apple in a friendly tone. They cooperate without difficulty when you tell them that playtime is over. They encounter the dog that barked at them last time and are able to remain calm, even though they feel afraid. And they can move through defensive emotions such as anger, sadness, and shame without them overwhelming him or "hijacking" their amygdala. In other words, the accelerator and the brake are in sync and cooperating with each other.

However, we know that this is not always the case, nor can we expect it to be. For a 7-year-old girl who has gone to her best friend's birthday party and sees other girls taking up all the attention of her dear friend, the experience that can make her feel overwhelmed, furious, and eager to yell at the first person who asks her what's wrong. In other words, the intensity of her emotions takes her out of her window of tolerance and moves her into what is known as the "red zone" or "hyperarousal zone," where "acute stress" is activated and the defense mechanism that is triggered is fight or flight. In this zone, your child's lower brain takes control of the four elements: body, cognition, behavior, and emotions. The most well-known behaviors in the red zone are usually the dreaded tantrums, screaming, pushing, biting, crying due to separation anxiety, etc. If you are a caregiver and have been responsible for at least one child, you will surely remember other manifestations of what it means to be in the red zone.

At other times, your child may become angry or very fearful, but instead of entering the red zone, the zone of hyperarousal, they descend into the blue zone, the zone of hypoarousal. In this zone, the defense mechanisms freeze or surrender. In this case, when faced with a situation that triggers defensive emotions such as anger, fear, sadness, or anxiety, the parasympathetic nervous system takes over, so instead of accelerating and setting the child in motion, it slows down so much that it seems as if the child has shut down. Behaviorally, the child may appear withdrawn, unwilling to interact with others, isolated, or persistently unable to speak or interact with anyone other than close family members. When we talk about simple and complex trauma, some of the symptoms children show have to do with the activation of their parasympathetic system being activated. Physically, when a child is hypoaroused, their heart rate slows down, as do their breathing rate and blood pressure. They may also have difficulty maintaining eye contact with others.

Many children diagnosed with anxiety disorders such as selective mutism, social anxiety, or agoraphobia tend to be in the blue zone of hypoarousal when they perceive that the situation they are experiencing has no way out, which often causes them to feel deeply afraid and in constant danger.

Neither children nor adults choose to be in one zone or another. Our autonomic nervous system is what "decides" which response is the most functional or adaptive according to the demands of the situation, based on how many times we have experienced that same situation and what we have learned from it that has been stored in its memory. Of course, it also has to do with the child's temperament and the adult's personality.

All children, whether anxious or not, have been in both the blue and red zones; we adults have too.

However, children who have gradually expanded their green zone by spending more and more time in it are more likely to overcome the disappointments, sadness, injustices, and situations that are part of life, with the functional belief that even in the midst of the storm, they can emerge transformed. Of course, they cannot achieve this alone. In reality, it is a call to caregivers; part of our job as parents is to help our children return to their green zone when we see them moving up toward the red zone or down toward the blue zone, so that we can help them gradually expand it through the different experiences they have in their daily lives.

8.3 Help your child deal with their anxiety and defensive emotions by talking and thinking about them

Learning to listen and validate our children's emotional world in an empathetic way is a fundamental part of parenting. The ability to listen to our children empathetically, that is, without judgment, but rather by tuning in to their emotional world and validating it, encourages the development of secure attachments and reduces the levels of stress our children experience as a result of the situations they encounter in their daily lives.

We understand ourselves by telling stories. When we have the opportunity to tell our own story, we are able to make sense of the experiences we have had. Talking and thinking about them allows us to organize them, place them in time, and see what we may not have been able to see at the time. But we cannot do this alone; we need the presence of another significant person, and in the case of children, this is imperative.

When a child experiences moments of distress, pain, or fear, they can become overwhelmed and their right hemisphere—which is responsible for emotions and feelings—can become overactive.

The right brain and lower brain experience a flood of intense emotions and bodily sensations that seem to plunge the child into chaos. In such cases, we, as caregivers, can help them engage their left hemisphere and the wisdom of their upper brain. Remember that the goal is to help and teach our children to experience their emotions, embrace them, and validate them, but without letting them take control of their lives. As we have already said, it is important to help them expand their green zone or window of tolerance. One of the best ways to foster this is by helping them talk and think about it.

"If we can carry out these tasks with our caregivers, the experience can be transformed into learning, as the resulting narrative will contain all the necessary material (properly translated) and generate appropriate beliefs about ourselves and our surroundings."[2]

One day, when my youngest son was 2 years old, he rode with me on a ride at a theme park in the city where we live: it was suitable for his age and height. In fact, we went there because he wanted to ride that particular ride, as it featured his favorite characters. Once it started moving and the distinctive sound of these rides could be heard, my son clung tightly to my arm and began to cry until the ride was over. After this experience, he didn't want to go on anything else during our stay at the park. When I saw my son "paralyzed" by fear, I remembered that, at that moment, his right hemisphere and lower brain were being overwhelmed by a flood of emotions and that the best thing I could do was help him talk and think about it by sitting down with him and telling him everything that had happened before we got on the ride and until we got off: "When we arrived at the park, we went running to get on your favorite ride. While we waited in line, I showed you the faces of the children who were having a great time with their parents, remember? You laughed and said you wanted to get on right away. Then it was our turn, we got into the car with your favorite picture on it and fastened our seatbelts. Then it started moving and we heard the loud noise it made, and you got scared, grabbed my arm, and started crying. Do you remember how I hugged you and kept saying, 'You're safe, you're secure, you're with me'? Then it stopped moving and making that noise, and I picked you up and we got off."

Since my 2-year-old son didn't have the words to tell me everything he was feeling, I helped him by describing what I saw in him as if I were a mirror, using the four elements: "Your face showed me that you were very scared, your eyes were closed, and your head was resting on my legs. Your heart was racing (body), because you thought we might fall (cognition), and then you started crying (behavior) because you were afraid (emotion)."

Why was it important to talk about it and think about it? Because when we do this, we help our children resignify their experience by integrating their brain hemispheres. "We want our children to be horizontally integrated, so that their left-brain logic can work well with their right-brain emotions. We also want them to be vertically integrated, so that the parts physically located in the upper part of their brain, which allow them to view their own actions in a reflective manner, work well with the lower parts, which are more related to instinct, visceral reactions, and survival."[3]

A few days later, my son continued to remember that episode and, in his own words, recounted it to me over and over again, and I continued to encourage and support him to do so every time he brought it up. This went on for three and a half months, as he recounted what had happened. Finally, he was able to reframe his experience, return to the park, and ride his favorite attraction, enjoying it as he had wanted to do from the beginning.

Allowing and encouraging children to talk and think about events that have overwhelmed them emotionally helps calm the traumatic and frightening emotions located in their right hemisphere and lower brain. Science confirms that naming what we are feeling reduces the activity of the emotional circuit triggered in the right hemisphere. As they put into words what happened and describe it in detail, they access the logic of their left hemisphere and the reflective capacity of their upper brain. It is as if, in some way, the upper brain says to the lower brain, "Calm down, it's over, you're alive, you're here right now and you're safe."

What happens when they don't want to talk or even think about it? This is also very common and happens when children are older. The fear, anxiety, or frustration they feel is so overwhelming that it makes it difficult for them to talk about it. In these cases, we must respect their feelings and their desire to remain silent. If we think it is appropriate, we can try to tell them what has happened, or what we think may have happened, and encourage them to add details. But if, even then, we see that they do not want to talk, then we must leave it for another time.

If we force them to talk when they don't want to, we can make them feel worse, just as this can happen to us. When we feel sad, angry, or anxious about something and someone insists that we tell them what's wrong even though we don't want to talk, even if their intentions are genuine, it can be upsetting for us.

We must always connect with our children's emotional world first, before attempting to redirect their behavior. In many cases, connecting means respecting their silence and simply accompanying them with our understanding; sometimes we accompany them by being by their side, and other times, simply by letting them know that we are physically available for them whenever they want us to be.

As a mother of three and a psychotherapist, I have also learned that very often the ideal time to talk and think about what has happened is in different contexts; for example, when we are having a snack, when we are in the car, when we are reading a story, or while we are playing with a puzzle or any other game. At these times, when the child and caregiver are calm, there is usually a greater willingness to talk and think about what has happened. In therapy sessions, we usually encourage children to draw what they feel if they don't want to talk, or to write down what has happened as if it were a story.

Whether immediately after the event or a few days later, what our children usually need when they experience something overwhelming is someone willing to help them put their emotional chaos into words; that is, to help them integrate their brain vertically and horizontally.

8.4 Five essential actions to reduce anxiety and stress in childhood: the CUIDAR technique

Nowadays, we talk a lot about the importance of taking care of ourselves. Talking about healthy living has become an almost essential topic in any setting. We have no doubt that encouraging the consumption of healthy foods in our children's diet is a responsibility that we must assume as caregivers.

Just as we take care of our children's physical health, it is our responsibility to take care of their mental and emotional health.

There are activities we can work on little by little to help our children integrate them into healthy lifestyle habits. In doing so, we are promoting balance and integration in our children's brains, as well as our own.

To make it easy to remember and meaningful in our work as caregivers, I wanted to use this acronym: *CUIDAR* ("*CARE*"), because caring sums up much of what we have discussed throughout the book. When we accompany, validate, support, and also invest time in teaching our children, we are caring for them. We care for our relationship with them; we care for their emotional world; we care for the construction of their own history, understanding that we are life coaches and that, as such, we are educating them for the moment and for life. *CUIDAR* is a reminder that this is precisely what much of our work as parents consists of.

Concentration: It is a distinctly human process that is acquired over time and requires the intervention of another person to develop. We are born with an immature brain that takes between 23 and 25 years to develop. We learn to concentrate because someone taught us how to do so. Rafa Guerrero, author of the book Cómo estimular el cerebro del niño (How to stimulate a child's brain), suggests different activities to stimulate our children's prefrontal cortex in order to help them develop their concentration. Among them, he suggests board games. They are a great alternative for this purpose. Intentionally dedicating time to playing Parcheesi, bingo, cards, or any other board game not only exercises the muscle of concentration, but is also an excellent way to nurture the relationship with our children, since most of these games involve four key elements: physical presence, eye contact, physical contact, and play. Other suggestions for developing concentration include reading a story together, doing Sudoku puzzles, word searches, and finding similarities and differences.

This is challenging, considering that today this type of game has lost the interest it held in other generations. Today, video games and activities that do not require mental effort often prevail. José Antonio Marina quotes[4] Zygmunt Bauman in one of his books: "More and more American children, and with increasing frequency, find the effort involved in eating an apple overwhelming: too much hard work for their jaws and teeth and, moreover, an excessive investment of time for the amount of pleasure obtained. These children also dislike having to peel an orange and prefer to drink packaged juice."

Use your hands: Put them to work! This is a literal expression for including manual activities in our children's daily lives. Help your children do tasks that involve using their hands. Some ideas could be: peeling potatoes, painting, kneading plasticine or clay, doing puzzles, making churros and balls and then crushing them with your index finger or thumb, planting seeds in the garden, building sandcastles… Crafts strengthen the gray matter. They help train patience and delay gratification, as you have to wait until the end to see the results.

This effort helps develop fine motor skills, encourage imagination and creativity, and allow children to learn sequencing. For these reasons and many more, it is important that we take a moment each day to do some of these activities with our children.

Inactivity: This word can give rise to the misconception of "wasting time." We are overwhelmed by the number of suggestions for how our children should make wise use of their time such as learning English, Chinese, German, robotics, piano, or math.

I am not against extracurricular classes; I consider them a great alternative and, as a mother of three, I am very grateful to have so many options available. What I find disproportionate is keeping our children so busy that our desire for them to make good use of their time takes away from their time to play, spend time with their friends, and get the sleep they need, or even leads us to sign them up for certain activities more on a whim than because our child really enjoys or needs that activity. We can encourage downtime by playing relaxing music and lying on the floor without any specific goal, simply enjoying the moment and feeling our breath come in and out.

Daily physical activity: Physical activity promotes physical growth and mental well-being in children and adults. When we exercise our bodies, we release dopamine, a neurotransmitter that helps us feel more energetic and emotionally balanced. Some options for physical activity at any time of day include cycling, skating, dancing at home, jumping rope, taking a walk around the neighborhood, or playing in the park. Various studies show that playing sports or taking time out of the day for physical activity supports concentration, learning, and memory, and also improves the quality of our sleep and rest.

Activities with friends: Let us not allow new technologies to "rob" us of our human need to share with others. We are social beings; we develop in relation to others. Sharing with others is not a desire, but an innate and necessary need for living. Intentionally set aside time for you and your child to share and bond with others. Having a picnic, hosting a sleepover, going hiking, meeting up with friends to make *pizza,* or simply getting together with your friends and your children's friends for the sake of enjoyment can be excellent ways to encourage socialization.

Rest: Rest is a fundamental need and not just a time of day when all activity ceases. Sleeping well and getting the necessary amount of sleep helps us to repair ourselves cognitively, emotionally, and physically. Have you ever had to stay up late for some reason and then found yourself unable to tolerate yourself the next day? When a child or anyone else does not get the amount of sleep they need, their learning and memory processes are disrupted. I liken getting a good night's sleep to the function of a cell phone charger: it recharges us with the energy we need to function. Therefore, make rest and sleep a cornerstone of your children's lives and your own. Avoid exposure to screens or any technological devices at least two hours before bedtime, gradually reduce physical activity, make sure dinner is light, and encourage bedtime rituals: a shower, dinner, reading a story, and sleep.

Various pediatric associations, such as the Spanish Pediatric Association and the American Academy of Sleep Medicine, recommend the following hours of sleep according to the child's age:

Age	*Hours of Sleep Needed*
Newborns to 2 years old	16–18 hours per day (including naps)
3–5	10–12 hours per day (including naps)
6–12 years	9–12 hours per day
13–18	8–10 hours per day

Notes

1 Porges, S. (2018). *Guía de bolsillo de la teoría polivagal. El poder transformador de sentirse seguro.* Barcelona: Editorial Eleftheria.
2 Aznárez, B. (2021), *El trauma psíquico es de todos. Rompe el silencio.* Edición: www.triunfacontulibro.com.
3 Siegel, D., and Bryson, T.P. (2012). *El cerebro del niño. 12 estrategias revolucionarias para cultivar la mente en desarrollo de tu hijo*. Barcelona: Alba.
4 Marina, J. (2019). *El cerebro infantil: la gran oportunidad* (5th ed.). Barcelona: Editorial Planeta.

References

Note: English translations and original English titles are given in square brackets following the Spanish title. Where a published English-language edition exists, its published English title has been used.

Alonso, M., Esteban, C., Gregoris, L., et al. (2012). *Máster en Inteligencia Emocional. Módulo V. Emociones Desadaptativas. Emocional.* [*Master's Degree in Emotional Intelligence. Module V. Maladaptive Emotions. Emotional*]. Valencia: Alfa Delta Digital.

Aznárez, B. (2020). *Psicoterapia breve con niños y adolescentes. El arte de entender, manejar, disfrutar y transformar la relación padres-hijos en terapia.* [*Brief Psychotherapy with Children and Adolescents. The Art of Understanding, Managing, Enjoying, and Transforming the Parent-Child Relationship in Therapy*]. Barcelona: Editorial Marcombo.

Aznárez, B. (2021). *El trauma psíquico es de todos. Rompe el silencio.* [*Psychological Trauma Affects Us All. Break the Silence*]. Edición: www.triunfacontulibro.com.

Barudy, J., and Dantagnan, M. (2005). *Los buenos tratos a la infancia. Parentalidad, apego y resiliencia.* [*Good Treatment of Children. Parenting, Attachment, and Resilience*]. Barcelona: Gedisa.

Bermejo, M. (2019). *Plantánimals. La emocipedia infantil.* [*Plantánimals. The Children's Emocipedia*]. Barcelona: Editorial Marcombo.

Bernal, M., and Lopera, J. (2002). *La culpa es de la vaca. Anécdotas, parábolas, fábulas y reflexiones sobre el liderazgo.* [*It's the Cow's Fault. Anecdotes, Parables, Fables, and Reflections on Leadership*]. Bogotá: Intermedio Editores Ltda.

Berne, E. (2014). *Más allá de juegos y guiones. Una selección de todas las obras del creador del Análisis Transaccional* [*Beyond Games and Scripts. A Selection of All the Works of the Creator of Transactional Analysis*]. Compiled by C. Steiner. Seville: Editorial Jeder.

Bowlby, J. (1989). *Una base segura: aplicaciones clínicas de la teoría del apego.* [*A Secure Base: Clinical Applications of Attachment Theory*]. Barcelona: Paidós Ibérica.

Cyrulnik, B. (2013). *Los patitos feos. La resiliencia. Una infancia infeliz no determina la vida.* [*The Ugly Ducklings. Resilience. An Unhappy Childhood Does Not Determine Your Life*]. Barcelona: Penguin Random House Grupo Editorial.

Dreikurs, R. (1991). *Children: The Challenge: The Classic Work on Improving Parent-Child Relations—Intelligent, Humane, and Eminently Practical.* New York, NY: Plume.

Edwards, G. (2011). *El triángulo dramático de Karpman. Cómo trascender los roles de perseguidor, salvador o víctima.* [*Karpman's Drama Triangle. How to Transcend the Roles of Persecutor, Rescuer, or Victim*] Móstoles: Gaia Ediciones.

Goleman, D. (1996). *Inteligencia emocional.* [*Emotional Intelligence.*] Barcelona: Editorial Kairós.

Guerrero, R. (2020a). *Cómo estimular el cerebro del niño. 100 ejercicios para potenciar la concentración, la atención, la memoria y otras funciones ejecutivas.* [*How to Stimulate the Child's Brain: 100 Exercises to Boost Concentration, Memory, and Other Executive Functions*] Madrid: Editorial Sentir.

Guerrero, R. (2020b). *Educar en el vínculo.* [*Educating through Bonding*] Barcelona: Plataforma Actual.

Marina, J. (2019). *El cerebro infantil: la gran oportunidad* [*The Child's Brain: The Great Opportunity*] (5th ed.). Barcelona: Editorial Planeta.

Mary, C., Blais-Rochette, C., Kokou-Kpolou, C., et al. (2021). "Prevalence of symptoms of depression, anxiety, insomnia, posttraumatic stress disorder, and psychological distress among populations affected by the COVID-19 pandemic: A systematic review and meta-analysis." *Psychiatry Research*, 295, pp. 1–16.

Núñez, C., and Valcárcel, R. (2013). *Emocionario. Di lo que sientes* [*Emotionary. Say What You Feel*]. Madrid: Palabras Aladas.

Orgiles, M., Morales, A., Delvecchio, E., et al. "Immediate psychological effects of the COVID-19 quarantine in youth from Italy and Spain". *PsyArXiv*; Apr. 2020 (cited April 23, 2020). Available at: https://osf.io/5bpfz

Osgood, K., Sheldon-Dean, H., and Kimball, H. (2021). *2021 Children's Mental Health Report: What We Know about the COVID-19 Pandemic's Impact on Children's Mental Health—and What We Don't Know*. New York, NY: Child Mind Institute.

Porges, S. (2018). *Guía de bolsillo de la teoría polivagal. El poder transformador de sentirse seguro* [*The Pocket Guide to the Polyvagal Theory: The Transformative Power of Feeling Safe*]. Barcelona: Editorial Eleftheria.

Seligman, M. (2016). *Niños optimistas* [*The Optimistic Child*]. Barcelona: Penguin Random House Grupo Editorial.

Siegel, D. J., and Bryson, T. P. (2012). *El cerebro del niño. 12 estrategias revolucionarias para cultivar la mente en desarrollo de tu hijo* [*The Whole-Brain Child: 12 Revolutionary Strategies to Nurture Your Child's Developing Mind*]. Barcelona: Alba.

Siegel, D. J., and Bryson, T. P. (2019). *Disciplina sin lágrimas. Una guía imprescindible para orientar y alimentar el desarrollo mental de tu hijo* [*No-Drama Discipline: The Whole-Brain Way to Calm the Chaos and Nurture Your Child's Developing Mind*]. Barcelona: Penguin Random House Grupo Editorial.

Siegel, D. J., and Bryson, T. P. (2020). *El poder de la presencia. Cómo la presencia de los padres moldea el cerebro de los hijos y configura las personas que llegarán a ser* [*The Power of Showing Up: How Parental Presence Shapes Who Our Kids Become and How Their Brains Get Wired*]. Barcelona: Alba.

Siegel, D. J., and Hartzell, M. (2019). *Ser padres conscientes. Un mejor conocimiento de nosotros mismos contribuye a un desarrollo integral de nuestros hijos* [*Parenting from the Inside Out: How a Deeper Self-Understanding Can Help You Raise Children Who Thrive*]. Barcelona: Ediciones La Llave.

UN Women. "The Shadow Pandemic: Violence against Women during COVID-19." Available at: https://www.unwomen.org/en/news/in-focus/in-focus-gender-equality-in-covid-19-response/violence-against-women-during-covid-19

UNICEF. (2018). *Operational Guidelines on Community-Based Mental Health and Psychosocial Support in Humanitarian Settings: Three-Tiered Support for Children and Families*. New York, NY: UNICEF. Available at: https://www.unicef.org/media/52171/file/Mental%20health%20and%20psychosocial%20support%20guidelines%202019%20.pdf

UNICEF Spain. (2020). *Salud mental e infancia en el escenario de la COVID-19. Propuestas de UNICEF España* [*Mental Health and Children in the Context of COVID-19. Proposals from UNICEF Spain*]. June 2020. Available at: https://www.unicef.es/publicacion/salud-mental-e-infancia-en-el-escenario-de-la-covid-19-propuestas-de-unicef-espana

van der Kolk, B. (2017). *El cuerpo lleva la cuenta. Cerebro, mente y cuerpo en la superación del trauma* [*The Body Keeps the Score: Brain, Mind, and Body in the Healing of Trauma*]. Barcelona: Eleftheria.

World Health Organization. (2022). "Mental health: Strengthening our response." June 17, 2022. Available at: https://www.who.int/es/news-room/fact-sheets/detail/mental-healthstrengthening-our-response

Index

For Product Safety Concerns and Information please contact our EU
representative GPSR@taylorandfrancis.com
Taylor & Francis Verlag GmbH, Kaufingerstraße 24, 80331 München, Germany

www.ingramcontent.com/pod-product-compliance
Lightning Source LLC
LaVergne TN
LVHW020831241026
850939LV00027B/401

* 9 7 8 1 0 4 1 2 8 0 4 3 9 *